THE MEDITERRANEAN DIET COOKBOOK

80 Easy, Delicious, and Healthy

30 MINUTE Recipes to Help You Lose Weight, Increase Your Energy, and Prevent Heart Disease, Stroke, and Diabetes

Gina Crawford

D1354089

Copyright © 2015 by Gina Crawford

Evita Publishing, PO Box 306, Station A, Vancouver Island, BC V9W 5B1 Canada

IMPORTANT

The information in this book reflects the author's research, experiences and opinions and is not intended to replace medical advice.

Before beginning this or any nutritional or exercise regimen, consult your physician to be sure it is appropriate for you. Ask for a physical stress test.

Table of Contents

Introduction

I truly believe that you are what you eat. If you eat well-balanced, nutritious meals made from natural whole foods then your body will thank you for it by performing at its best.

The Mediterranean diet doesn't restrict or exclude foods rather it encourages the consumption of a variety of foods in moderation. This makes it both a friendly and effective diet because it won't give you the "I feel so deprived" diet blues shortly after starting it.

Fresh fruits, vegetables and whole grains are a popular staple on the Mediterranean diet. Consuming fish and seafood weekly for their omega-3 benefits is important and making olive oil a primary source of monounsaturated fat is a necessary component of the Mediterranean diet. Consuming dairy, poultry, red wine and sweets are also important characteristics of the Mediterranean diet.

In this book, I have included 80 of my favorite 30 MINUTE Mediterranean diet recipes for breakfast, lunch and dinner PLUS... salad recipes, side dishes, snacks, dressings, dips and sauces.

Each recipe reflects the dietary eating habits of the people of Crete in the 1950's and 60's.

When you eat a well-balanced diet and exercise regularly as the Mediterranean diet suggests, you will lose weight, revitalize your energy, and prevent heart disease, diabetes, arthritis, Alzheimer's, Parkinson's, and certain kinds of cancer.

The Mediterranean diet also helps to lower cholesterol and blood pressure, and improve brain and eye health.

My hope is that the variety of delicious recipes that I have included in this cookbook will allow you to dive right into making the Mediterranean way of eating a lifestyle!

Enjoy!

A Note About Measurements in This Book

For my UK friends: In order to get the most accurate measurements for each recipe, I highly recommend purchasing a set of North American measuring cups (a liquid measure and a dry measure). You can purchase a set of each online. This will make cooking these delicious recipes a breeze!

Chapter 1

What is the Mediterranean Diet?

"The doctor of the future will no longer treat the human frame with drugs, but rather will cure and prevent disease with nutrition."
Thomas Edison

The Mediterranean diet isn't actually a "diet." Yes, it can help you lose weight and improve your health but it's really more of a lifestyle. It's a way of eating that can keep you healthy for a long time and provide all the nutrients you need to live life to the fullest.

The Mediterranean diet is based on the traditional dietary patterns of the countries that border the Mediterranean Sea, such as Greece, Spain, Israel, Southern Italy and France. It gained widespread popularity in the west during the 1990's and since then has become one of the most well-respected diets, particularly for its heart-health and longevity benefits.

There are 21 countries that border the Mediterranean Sea and though their diets, culture, agriculture, ethnic background and economy vary there are common dietary patterns that they share. These common patterns have become characteristic of what we call the Mediterranean diet.

The most authentic version of the Mediterranean diet is based on the typical dietary patterns of the people of Crete (the largest Greek island) during the 1950's and 60's.

Characteristics of the Mediterranean diet

High consumption of food from plant sources: fruits, vegetables, legumes, nuts, seeds, breads, grains, potatoes, unrefined cereals

Olive oil is the primary source of monounsaturated fat replacing other oils and fats (including margarine and butter)

Moderate consumption of red wine, fish, dairy (primarily yogurt and cheese), poultry, eggs and sweets

Low consumption of red meat

Zero to four eggs consumed weekly

Substitution of salts for spices such as basil and oregano

Fresh fruit as the typical dessert

Exercise daily

Replace salt with herbs and spices

Why choose the Mediterranean Diet?

The Mediterranean diet is easy to adapt to your lifestyle. Unlike many diets that involve increasing your intake of certain vitamins and minerals, the Mediterranean diet is different in that it allows you to eat a wide variety of foods.

Also, the foods on the Mediterranean diet are foods that you already eat fairly regularly so adapting to a Mediterranean way of eating won't involve any drastic changes.

Chapter 2

A Brief History of the Mediterranean Diet

The origins of the Mediterranean diet date back to the Middle Ages in which the upper-class ancient Romans (modeling Greek tradition) would regularly consume wine, bread, olive oil, vegetables, fruit and cheese and an abundance of fish, various seafood and little red meat.

The health benefits of the Mediterranean diet were discovered by American scientist Ancel Benjamin Keys who avidly studied the influence of diet on health. His studies on the Mediterranean diet were the first to reveal a correlation between cardiovascular disease and diet.

During the 1950's Ancel Keys was shocked that people in the poorest small towns in Southern Italy were much healthier than the wealthy people in New York. Keys felt that this was a result of their diet. He went on to investigate and attempt to validate his belief by focusing his studies on the foods that were being consumed in these populations.

The Seven Countries Study

In 1958, he and Paul Dudley White the world's leading cardiologist at the time started the Seven Countries Study. This was a long running study (over 50 years) that documented the relationship between diet, lifestyle, stroke and cardiovascular disease in seven different countries of the world. It included cross-sectional studies that aimed to prove that the nutritional value of the Mediterranean diet contributed to a healthier body and longevity for the populations that adopted the Mediterranean way of eating.

Keys and White along with the support of researchers in each of the seven countries involved in the study, compiled data of over twelve thousand middle-aged men from the United States, Italy, Japan, Greece, Finland, the Netherlands, and Yugoslavia.

The findings of this study proved that populations that adopted a Mediterranean diet had low levels of cholesterol in their blood and a low percentage of cardiovascular disease.

The healthiest ranking area of the study was Crete. Cretan men had the most positive cardiovascular test results as a result of their diet and exercise patterns.

Scientific proof of the benefits of the Mediterranean diet

Keys studies started a flood of scientific research that looked at the correlation between chronic diseases and dietary habits. Many clinical trials and studies have proven that the Mediterranean way of eating reduces the risk of metabolic syndrome and cardiovascular disease.

Studies have also proven that adhering to a Mediterranean diet increases high density lipoprotein (HDL), decreases blood pressure, triglycerides, blood glucose levels and abdominal circumference.

Researchers continue to run new tests on the Mediterranean diet even today as they define the diets effects on the human body in further detail. New studies regularly appear in leading scientific journals supporting the health benefits of the Mediterranean diet.

The variety of test and clinical studies that have been and continue to be performed include tests on lengthened life span, improved brain function, preventing chronic diseases, fighting certain cancers, lowering heart disease, lowering blood pressure, reducing high cholesterol levels, preventing diabetes, promoting weight loss, alleviating depression, Alzheimer's, Parkinson's, rheumatoid arthritis and promoting eye health, better breathing, healthier babies and improved fertility.

Every one of the listed items above has a clinical report written about the Mediterranean diet and its positive effects on each health challenge. No other diet has as much documented proof of its effectiveness as the Mediterranean diet.

For more information on how to apply the Mediterranean diet to your life, check out my Mediterranean Diet for Beginners book on Amazon.

Chapter 3

Breakfast

Start your day the Mediterranean way with healthy, nutritious meals that will give you a boost of energy for living each day to the fullest!

Quinoa with Cinnamon and Chia Seeds

Quinoa, pronounced "KEEN-wah," can be found at your local grocery store or health food store. Quinoa acts like a grain, tastes like a grain but is not a grain or oat. It is actually part of the spinach, Swiss chard, and beet family. The part that we eat is the seed. Though it is cooked like rice, it is gluten-free. Quinoa is considered a complete protein because it contains all nine essential amino acids. It is also rich in fiber, iron, magnesium, manganese, riboflavin, and lysine.

Serves 4

Ingredients

Quinoa.....1/2 cup, uncooked

Unsweetened vanilla almond milk.....1 cup

Raisins.....2 tablespoons

Cinnamon.....1 teaspoon

Vanilla extract.....1/2 teaspoon

Chia seeds.....1/2 tablespoon

Maple syrup

Directions

Rinse the quinoa and cook it according to the package instructions.

In a small sauce pan, combine the quinoa and the unsweetened almond milk and bring it to a boil. Add half teaspoon vanilla extract and one teaspoon cinnamon. Reduce the heat to simmer and cook for about fifteen minutes or until the liquid has been absorbed by the quinoa. Stir often.

To serve, place some quinoa into a bowl and top with chia seeds, raisins, and maple syrup.

Whole Wheat Couscous with Apricots and Currants

Whole-wheat couscous is made from the whole grains found in durum flour. Durum wheat is high in protein and low in fat. Couscous is a great source of dietary fiber and iron. Fiber stabilizes blood sugar levels and keeps you feeling full. (Pronounced Koose Koose)

Serves 4

Ingredients

Low-fat milk..... 3 cups

Cinnamon stick.....1 - 2-inches

Whole wheat couscous.....1 cup, uncooked

Dried apricots.....1/2 cup, chopped

Dried currants.....1/4 cup

Dark brown sugar.....4 teaspoons for couscous - 2 teaspoons divided for topping

Salt.....1 teaspoon

Olive oil.....4 teaspoons, divided

Directions

Pour the low fat milk into a large saucepan then add the cinnamon stick. Cook over medium heat until small bubbles form. Do not boil.

Remove the milk from the heat. Stir in the apricots, currents, couscous, brown sugar, and salt.

Cover with a tight fitting lid for fifteen minutes.

Remove the cinnamon stick. Divide the couscous into four bowls.

Top each dish with one teaspoon of olive oil and half a teaspoon of brown sugar. Serve immediately.

Vegetable Omelet with Fennel

A vegetable omelet is extremely versatile. You can add any combination of vegetables that you like and it will taste great every time! Be creative and change things up in this recipe as often as you like!

Serves 4

Ingredients

Eggs.....6

Fennel bulb.....2 cups, thinly sliced

Roma tomato.....1 diced

Green brine-cured olives.....1/4 cup, pitted and chopped

Artichoke hearts.....1/4 cup marinated in water, rinsed, drained and chopped

Goat cheese.....1/2 cup, crumbled

Fresh dill, basil or parsley.....2 tablespoons, chopped

Extra virgin olive oil.....1 tablespoon

Salt and pepper.....to taste

Directions

Preheat the oven to 325 degrees.

In a skillet, heat the olive oil over medium high heat and sauté the fennel for five minutes.

Add the artichokes, tomato, and olives to the pan. Sauté for another three minutes or until the artichokes soften.

In a large bowl, whisk the six eggs, salt, and pepper together.

Pour the whisked egg mixture into the skillet over the vegetables and stir for a couple of minutes.

Sprinkle the crumbled goat cheese on top and place into oven. Bake for five minutes. Check to see if the eggs are cooked through by inserting a knife or fork through the center. It should come out clean of any liquid.

Remove from oven and allow the dish to set for one minute. Cut into four wedges.

Top with dill, basil or parsley and serve.

Mediterranean Breakfast Scramble with Potato, Olives and Ricotta Cheese

Ricotta cheese is a great source of protein. It is available in regular, fat-free and light varieties so you can indulge in this delicious Mediterranean diet breakfast knowing that your calorie intake is low!

Serves 4

Ingredients

New potatoes.....3 medium, thinly sliced

Red bell pepper....1/4 diced

Black olives.....8 sliced

Fresh parsley.....1/4 cup, chopped

Ricotta cheese.....1/4 cup

Eggs.....6

Whole grain bread.....4 slices

Extra virgin olive oil.....4 teaspoons

Pepper.....1/2 teaspoon

Salt.....1/2 teaspoon

Directions

Heat a large non-stick skillet over medium high heat. Add the olive oil.

While the oil is heating up, wash and thinly slice the potatoes then add them to the heated skillet. Sauté for fifteen minutes or until the potatoes turn golden brown. Add the red bell pepper and olives. Cook for an additional four minutes until the bell pepper starts to soften.

In a medium bowl whisk the eggs, parsley and ricotta cheese together.

Pour the egg mixture over the potato mixture and stir throughout the cooking time until the eggs firm up but not to the point of turning dry, about three minutes.

Add salt and pepper to taste.

Serve with whole grain bread slices, lightly toasted and brushed with olive oil. Yum!

Cinnamon Quinoa with Pistachios, Pomegranate, and Dried Apricots

Start the day with a terrific dish of quinoa, dried fruits, and nuts. Quinoa provides anti-inflammatory nutrients and antioxidants. It also helps lower the risk of cardiovascular disease.

Serves 4

Ingredients

Quinoa.....1 cup

Low-fat milk.....2 cups

Pistachio nuts.....1 ½ cups, unsalted and roasted

Pomegranate seeds.....1/4 cup

Ground cinnamon.....1/4 teaspoon

Allspice.....1/4 teaspoon

Apricots..... 1/2 cup, chopped

Sugar.....2 teaspoons

Directions

Dried fruit and nuts preparation:

Preheat the oven to 350 degrees.

Spread the pistachio nuts on a baking sheet and bake for several minutes or until lightly toasted. Remove from the oven and cool.

In a bowl, add the pomegranate seeds, pistachio nuts, cinnamon, allspice, sugar, and chopped apricots. Stir until the ingredients are well mixed.

Quinoa Preparation:

In a medium saucepan warm the quinoa then slowly add the two cups of low-fat milk while stirring.

Reduce the heat and cover. Simmer for fifteen minutes. Stir quinoa half way through the simmering period, about seven minutes.

Plating:

Spoon the quinoa into bowls. Add the dried fruit and nut mixture over top. Serve immediately. Enjoy!

Mediterranean Breakfast Wrap with Spinach and Fresh Basil

Feel free to experiment with this recipe and add whatever vegetables you like.

Makes 2 wraps

Ingredients

Eggs.....4 large

Yellow onion.....1/4 cup

Sweet red pepper.....1/4 cup

Tomato.....1 small, chopped

Fresh baby spinach.....1/2 cup, torn

Fresh basil....1 teaspoon, chopped

Whole wheat tortillas.....2 (7-8 inches)

Low-fat feta-cheese.....1 ounce, crumbled

Extra virgin olive oil.....3 tablespoons

Salt.....1/8 teaspoon

Pepper....1/4 teaspoon

Directions

Heat the oil in a non-stick pan. Add the onion then the sweet pepper. Cook the onion over medium heat until the onion is translucent. Add the eggs and fresh basil. Let the eggs set.

Place the baby spinach and tomato in the centre of the whole wheat tortilla. Top with the egg mixture and feta cheese. Fold and serve. :o)

Plum Tomato and Artichoke Breakfast Delight

Artichokes support digestive health and assist in lowering bad cholesterol and increasing good cholesterol. They also minimize irregular bowel symptoms and reduce heartburn. If you have gallbladder disease, consult your health care provider before eating the artichoke leaves or extracts as they could stimulate gallbladder contractions.

Serves 4

Ingredients

Artichoke hearts.....1/2 cup

Ripe plum tomato.....1/2 cup, chopped

Fresh basil leaves.....4 - 6 tablespoons

Feta cheese.....1/4 cup, crumbled

Eggs.....6

Whole-wheat pita pocket rounds.....2

Hot sauce.....1 teaspoon

Extra virgin olive oil.....2 tablespoons

Salt and pepper.....to taste

Directions

Add the artichoke hearts, chopped tomatoes, fresh basil leaves, and crumbled feta cheese to a large bowl. Set aside.

In a small bowl, beat the six eggs until they are evenly colored and bubbly.

Pour the beaten eggs into the large bowl of artichoke hearts, tomatoes, basil, and feta cheese. Stir while folding the ingredients into the egg mixture. Evenly coat the ingredients with the egg.

Heat the olive oil in a pan on medium heat. Add the artichoke egg mixture to the pan. Stir and cook through, about five minutes.

When the egg mixture is cooked, place it into the pita and add hot sauce.

Season with salt and pepper.

Cheesy Basil and Feta Mediterranean Scramble

Feta is a white, brined curd cheese typically made in Greece from sheep's milk or a combination of sheep's milk and goat's milk. North American Feta cheese is made from cow's milk. Feta cheese tends to be a little high in sodium. You can reduce the sodium content by soaking it in water before using it. It's also interesting to note that sheep's milk contains higher levels of nutrients than cow's milk.

Serves 6

Ingredients

Eggs.....10

Dried Basil.....1/2 teaspoon

Red bell pepper.....1 small finely chopped

Sweet onion.....1 small finely chopped

Feta cheese.....2 tablespoons crumbled, low sodium, low fat

Whole-wheat bread slices.....6 toasted

Extra virgin olive oil.....1 ½ tablespoons

Directions

Heat the olive oil in a medium sized skillet over medium heat.

In a medium bowl add the dried basil, some black pepper and the eggs. Whisk until well blended.

In the skillet that contains the olive oil add the red pepper and onion. Sauté until the onion is tender and opaque.

Pour eggs, basil and black pepper mixture over the red pepper and onion mixture. Allow the egg to start setting and stir occasionally until the eggs cook through.

Sprinkle crumbled feta cheese over top.

Plate the eggs and serve with toasted whole-wheat bread.

Mediterranean Pizza Omelet

Passata sauce is a jarred tomato sauce that is as thick as a canned paste. Passata includes fiber, vitamins A, B6, C, E, K, riboflavin, niacin, pantothenic acid, magnesium, phosphorus, iron, potassium, copper and manganese.

Serves 4

Ingredients

Eggs.....8

Oregano.....1 teaspoon

Extra virgin olive oil.....1 tablespoon

Tomato Passata sauce.....4 tablespoons (Tomato or pizza sauce with the consistency of a tomato paste)

Black olives.....10 pitted and sliced

Cheddar cheese.....2 cups shredded

Salt.....pinch

Pepper.....pinch

Directions

Heat a skillet on medium-low heat. Add olive oil.

In a medium bowl add eggs, oregano and pinch of salt and pepper. Whisk together.

Pour eggs into the heated olive oil and tip the pan around until the eggs set.

Stir occasionally until the eggs puff up, about four minutes.

Pour the passata sauce over the set eggs then add the sliced olives over the sauced area. Sprinkle the cheddar cheese over top. Place a lid on the skillet for two minutes. Remove from the heat source. Slice and serve immediately.

Spinach Supreme Omelet with Ham and Cheese

On the Mediterranean diet, breakfast, lunch, dinner and snacking can all include heart-healthy vegetables like spinach. Spinach is a nutrient-rich food that is high in vitamins, minerals and phytonutrients. It is a leafy green vegetable that is a great source of vitamin K, magnesium, iron, vitamin A, folate, vitamin B2, vitamin B6, vitamin C, potassium, protein, vitamin E, zinc, phosphorus, fiber, and copper, selenium and omega-3 fatty acids.

Serves 2

Ingredients

Eggs.....2

Water.....2 tablespoons

Italian cheese blend.....1/4 cup shredded

Baby spinach.....1/4 cup

Low fat ham.....1/4 cup finely chopped

Extra virgin olive oil.....1 teaspoon

Salt and pepper.....to taste

Directions

In a small bowl add the eggs and water and whisk.

Heat a nonstick skillet over medium-high heat. Add the oil. Tilt the pan in order to coat it evenly with the oil.

Add the whisked eggs to the skillet and tilt the pan around in a circular motion so that the eggs cover the bottom of the pan evenly. The outer edges of the egg should begin to set immediately.

When the egg sets, add the shredded Italian cheese blend, baby spinach and finely chopped ham to one side of the eggs.

Use a spatula and flip the empty portion of the egg over top of the cheesy portion to make the omelet.

Transfer the omelet to a plate. Add salt and pepper to taste. Serve.

Granola with Greek Yogurt, Rosemary Honey and Blueberries

There are a number of differences between Greek yogurt and regular yogurt. Both start out with the same ingredients – bacterial cultures and milk. Lactic acid is produced when the bacteria ferment the lactose found in the milk. When fermentation is complete, the yogurt goes through a straining process that strains off the liquid whey.

Regular yogurt is only strained twice whereas Greek yogurt is strained three times. The more that yogurt is strained the less liquid it retains. This is why Greek yogurt has a thick consistency compared to regular yogurt. This also makes Greek yogurt more concentrated and higher in protein than regular yogurt. Greek yogurt contains double the amount of protein than regular yogurt. This provides a fuller feeling for a longer period of time which cuts down on snacking between meals. Greek yogurt also contains half the amount of sodium than regular yogurt.

Serves 4

Ingredients

Rolled Oats.....3 cups

Walnuts.....1/4 cup

Almonds.....1/4 cup

Cashews.....1/4 cup

Coconut..... 2 tablespoons shredded

Maple syrup.....1/4 cup

Vanilla extract.....1 teaspoon

Light sesame oil.....1/4 cup

Dried apricots.....1/2 cup

Dried cranberries.....1/2 cup

Greek style yogurt.....2 cups

Rosemary honey.....1/2 cup

Blueberries.....1 cup

Directions

Preheat the oven to 325 degrees

In a large bowl, stir together the oats, walnuts, almonds, cashews, coconut, dried apricots and dried cranberries.

In a small bowl, stir together the maple syrup, sesame oil and vanilla extract. Drizzle over the oats and nut mixture and stir.

Transfer the oats and nuts to a rimmed cookie sheet and spread evenly. Place into the oven and bake. Stir after several minutes then continue to bake until the oats turn brown., about twenty minutes.

The granola should feel dry. It becomes crispy as it cools. You can store it in an airtight container up to a week for additional uses.

Divide the yogurt into four bowls. Top each bowl of yogurt with a quarter cup of granola.

Sprinkle a quarter cup of blueberries on top of the granola. Drizzle the rosemary honey on top of the blueberries. Serve immediately.

Chapter 4

Lunch

In Mediterranean countries it is common for shop owners to close their stores at midday, go home, have lunch with their kids, take a restful nap then re-open their stores later that afternoon.

The Mediterranean people understand the importance of slowing down. This is an important aspect of the Mediterranean diet.

Mediterranean Chicken Gyros

Gyros are very popular in Greece. They are a very versatile food because you can put almost anything that you like in them. The meat can be changed up to pork or lamb, the vegetables can be replaced with whatever you like and the sauce can be replaced with a nice garlic or tzatziki sauce. A nice, quick Mediterranean diet meal!

Serves 4

Ingredients

Chicken breast.....1/2 pound, boneless, skinless cut into ½ inch strips

Greek yogurt.....1/3 cup plain

Pita bread or Gyro bread.....2

Cucumber.....1/2 cup chopped

Red onion.....1/2 small, sliced

Lemon.....1/4 cup lemon juice

Garlic.....2 teaspoons minced, divided

Dill weed.....1/4 teaspoon

Ground mustard.....1/2 teaspoon

Dried oregano.....1/2 teaspoon

Romaine lettuce.....6 leaves

Tomato.....2 chopped

Extra virgin olive oil.....1/4 cup

Olive oil cooking spray

Directions

Combine the olive oil, lemon juice, ground mustard, 1 teaspoon of garlic and oregano in a large Ziploc bag. Add the chicken and turn the bag to distribute the marinade. Refrigerate for twenty minutes.

In a small bowl combine the yogurt, cucumber, dill weed and remaining garlic. After twenty minutes, remove the chicken from the bag and discard the marinade.

Spray a non-stick skillet with cooking spray and sauté the chicken for seven minutes. Place each pita on a plate. Spoon half the chicken on one pita and half on the other pita. Top with the red onion, cucumber mixture, lettuce and tomato. Fold each pita in half and serve. Yum!

Greek Salad

Black olives contain healthy unsaturated fat, calcium, fiber and vitamin A. The unsaturated fat reduces your risk of heart disease and if eaten regularly aids in lowering cholesterol levels as well as neutralizing free radicals that can lead to cancer.

Serves 6

Ingredients

Romaine lettuce.....1 head rinsed, dried, and chopped

Red onion.....1 thinly sliced

Black olives.....1 can pitted (6 ounces)

Green bell pepper.....1 chopped

Red bell pepper.....1 chopped

Tomatoes......2 large chopped

Cucumber.....1 sliced

Feta cheese.....1 cup crumbled

Lemon.....1 juiced

Extra virgin olive oil.....6 tablespoons

Dried oregano.....1 teaspoon

Ground black pepper, to taste

Directions

In a large bowl, combine the chopped bell peppers, crumbled feta cheese, sliced cucumbers, pitted-black olives, thinly sliced red onions, chopped tomatoes, and chopped Romaine lettuce.

In a smaller bowl, whisk together the black pepper, lemon juice, oregano and olive oil to make the dressing.

Pour the dressing over the salad, toss and serve immediately.

Garbanzo Chicken Salad with Feta and Fresh Basil

Three ounces of skinless chicken breast contains 27 grams of protein. Protein is an important building block of heart tissue, skeletal tissue, muscular tissue and the smooth muscle in the intestines. Chicken is also a great source of vitamin B3, B6 and selenium.

Serves 4

Ingredients

Chicken breast.....9 ounces, cooked and chopped

Garbanzo beans.....15 ounce can rinsed and drained

Baby spinach.....2 cups, rinsed

Feta cheese.....1/3 cup, crumbled

Greek yogurt..... ½ cup plain, fat-free

Cucumber.....1 cup, seeded

Green onions.....1/2 cup chopped

Fresh basil.....1/4 cup chopped

Garlic.....2 cloves, minced

Lemon.....4 wedges

Salt..... 1/4 teaspoon

Black pepper.....to taste

Pita chips or pita pockets

Directions

In a large bowl combine the cooked chicken breast, garbanzo beans, seeded cucumber, chopped green onion, chopped fresh basil, yogurt, garlic and salt.

Stir ingredients together gently then slowly fold in the rinsed baby spinach leaves.

Add crumbled feta cheese over top and pepper to taste. Serve immediately with pita chips or use pita pockets and make a sandwich.

Broiled Spanish Mackerel

Spanish Mackerel is a very tasty and healthy fish. In Japanese it is called *aji* which is the same as the word "taste" in Japanese. It got its name for its good taste. Spanish Mackerel is one of the richest sources of omega-3 fatty acids.

Serves 6

Ingredients

Spanish mackerel fillets.....6 - 3 ounces each

Extra virgin olive oil..... 1/4 cup split

Paprika.....1/2 teaspoon

Lemon.....2 for 12 slices

Salt.....1 teaspoon

Pepper.....1 teaspoon

Directions

Preheat the oven broiler and set the rack about six inches from the heat.

Lightly grease a baking dish with half the olive oil coating the bottom of the dish.

Rub both sides of Spanish mackerel with the remaining olive oil. Place skin side down on the prepared baking dish.

Season each fillet with salt, pepper and paprika. Top each with two lemon slices.

Bake fillets under the broiler for five to seven minutes or until the fish flakes. Serve immediately.

Sun-Dried Tomato Pesto

For a delicious meal, serve this recipe over some bow tie angel hair pasta or cheese ravioli. The pesto can also be used as a dip with Melba toast, corn tortillas, mozzarella sticks or any item you enjoy dipping into a pesto based sauce. Sun- dried tomatoes offer a rich source of vitamins and minerals that help maintain healthy bones, tissue, energy production, iron, manganese, copper, phosphorus as well as vitamins A, B5, B9, C, K and niacin.

Makes 2 ½ cups

Ingredients

Sun-dried tomatoes.....4 ounces

Fresh basil.....2 tablespoons chopped

Fresh parsley.....2 tablespoons chopped

Garlic.....1 tablespoon chopped

Pine nuts.....1/4 cup chopped

White onion.....3 tablespoons chopped

Balsamic vinegar.....1/4 cup

Tomato paste.....1 tablespoon

Tomatoes.....1/3 cup crushed

Red wine.....1/4 cup

Extra virgin olive oil.....1/2 cup

Parmesan cheese.....1/2 cup grated

Salt.....1 teaspoon

Pepper......to taste

Directions

Place the sun-dried tomatoes in a bowl with warm water for five minutes until rehydrated and tender.

In a food processor or blender combine the rehydrated sun dried tomatoes, basil, parsley, garlic, pine nuts and onions. Process until well blended.

Add balsamic vinegar, crushed tomatoes, tomato paste and red wine.

Process again until well blended.

Stir in olive oil and parmesan cheese.

Add salt and pepper to taste.

Roasted Bell Pepper and Artichoke Pasta Salad

Farfalle is the Italian equivalent for bow tie pasta. Farfalle is derived from the word farfalla which means butterfly in Italian.

Serves 4

Ingredients

Farfalle.....8 ounces, multi-grain

Artichoke hearts.....1 can (13.5 ounces) in water, drained and chopped

Mozzarella cheese.....8 ounces, partly skimmed, shredded

Roasted bell peppers.....1/4 cup, bottled, chopped

Peas.....1/2 cup, frozen

Fresh parsley.....1/4 cup chopped

Lemon.....1 zest and juice

Extra virgin olive oil.....2 teaspoons

Directions

Cook the farfalle according to the directions omitting any salt or added fats.

While the pasta cooks, combine the lemon zest, lemon juice and olive oil in a large bowl then whisk.

Add artichoke hearts, bell pepper, cheese and parsley then toss to combine.

Place peas in colander when the pasta is finished. Drain the pasta over the peas in the colander. Shake well but do not run water over them.

Add pasta and peas to the large bowl with the other ingredients. Toss well until thoroughly combined. Serve warm or at room temperature.

Seafood Couscous Paella

In Spanish, Saffron is called "zafran." Saffron is a spice that comes from the Crocus Sativus flower also known as saffron crocus. Saffron is considered the Lamborghini of spices. Why? Because it is cultivated and harvested by hand and it's extremely expensive. The reason it costs so much is because of the labor that's involved and because it often takes 75,000 saffron blossoms to create one pound of saffron spice. Saffron is very thread like because it is made from the thread-like (dried stigmas) of the flower.

Serves 2

Ingredients

Extra-virgin Olive oil.....2 teaspoons

Onion.....1 medium chopped

Garlic clove.....1 minced

Dried thyme.....1/2 teaspoon

Fennel seed.....1/2 teaspoon

Saffron threads.....pinch

Tomatoes.....1 cup diced

Vegetable broth.....1/4 cup

Bay scallops.....4 ounces tough muscle removed

Shrimp.....4 ounces medium peeled and deveined

Whole-wheat couscous.....1/2 cup

Freshly ground pepper.....1/4 teaspoon

Directions

Heat the olive oil in a medium saucepan over medium heat. Add the onion and cook for a few minutes until the onions turn opaque. Add minced garlic, dried thyme, fennel seed, salt, freshly ground pepper, crumbled saffron and vegetable broth. Cook for twenty minutes. Stir as the pot comes to a simmer. Cover and reduce heat to simmer an additional two minutes.

Wash the medium shrimp and bay scallops. Add shrimp and bay scallops to the simmering pot and stir to mix. Increase the heat back to medium and cook for an additional three minutes. Stir in the couscous and tomatoes. Turn the heat off. Put the lid back on the skillet and let the pot simmer for ten minutes. Transfer to a serving bowl and serve immediately.

Mediterranean Creamy Panini

Panino is the Italian word for a small bread roll or at times a sandwich.

Panini is the name that Europeans and Americans have given to a pressed or toasted sandwich. Panini's can be made of any type of bread as long as it is pressed and toasted.

Serves 4

Ingredients

Whole grain bread.....8 slices

Romaine lettuce.....8 leaves

Black olives.....2 tablespoons, pitted and chopped

Zucchini.....1 small, thinly sliced

Tomato.....1 sliced

Provolone cheese.....4 slices

Roasted red peppers.....1 jar, drained and sliced

Bacon.....8 slices, cooked

Fresh basil.....1/4 cup chopped

Homemade Mayonnaise.....1/4 cup

Extra virgin olive oil.....1 tablespoon

Homemade mayo:

Makes 3/4 cups of mayo

Egg.....1 large, yolk only

Lemon.....1 – juice only, 1 ½ teaspoons

White wine vinegar.....1 teaspoon

Dijon mustard.....1/4 teaspoon

Olive oil.....3/4 cup

Combine all the ingredients in a medium bowl. Whisk until blended.

Add a quarter cup of the olive oil to the mixture a few drops at a time. Slowly add the remaining half cup of olive oil whisking constantly.

Cover and put in the refrigerator. Keep chilled.

Directions

In a medium skillet on medium heat, cook the bacon until it's done. Move to a plate with paper towel on it to reduce fat drippings.

In a small bowl combine the mayonnaise with one tablespoon of olive oil. Stir. Add finely chopped black olives and basil to mayonnaise mixture and stir.

If you have a whole loaf of whole grain bread, use a breadboard and slice eight pieces of bread from the loaf on a diagonal slant.

Spread the mayonnaise mixture on each slice of bread. Add two slices of tomato, sliced zucchini, peppers, provolone, two bacon strips, one lettuce leaf and cover with another piece of bread mayonnaise side down toward the ingredients. Repeat three times to make other sandwiches.

Heat a large skillet to medium and place the sandwiches in the skillet to brown the bread, about five minutes each side.

Cut the sandwiches in half and serve immediately.

Mediterranean Halibut Sandwiches

Halibut is as nutritious as salmon when it comes to omega-3's and general nutrients. The human body cannot produce omega-3's so we must obtain polyunsaturated fatty acids from sources outside of our bodies. Omega-3 fatty acids can be found in cold-water fish like halibut, salmon, mackerel, sardines, tuna and herring. We can also get them from flaxseed, soybeans, pumpkin seeds, canola oil, and walnuts. Omega-3's lower triglycerides, blood pressure and inflammation and improve vascular functions. They also increase our metabolism.

Serves 4

Ingredients

Extra virgin olive oil cooking spray

Halibut fillets.....2 - 6 ounces each, skinned

Extra virgin olive oil.....2 teaspoons divided

Ciabatta bread.....1 loaf, (14 ounces) ends trimmed, split horizontally down the middle

Garlic clove.....1 halved

Homemade mayonnaise.....1/4 cup

Sun dried tomatoes.....1/4 cup chopped

Fresh basil.....1/4 cup chopped

Capers.....1 tablespoon drained and mashed

Lemon zest.....1 large

Arugula..... 2 cups

Black pepper.....to taste

Directions

Homemade mayonnaise:

Makes 3/4 cups of mayo

Egg.....1 large, yolk only

Lemon.....1 – juice only, 1 ½ teaspoons

White wine vinegar.....1 teaspoon

Dijon mustard.....1/4 teaspoon

Olive oil.....3/4 cup

Combine all the ingredients in a medium bowl. Whisk until blended.

Add a quarter cup of olive oil to the mixture a few drops at a time. Slowly add the remaining half cup of olive oil whisking constantly. Cover and put in the refrigerator. Keep chilled.

Halibut sandwiches:

Preheat the oven to 450 degrees. Use a small baking dish and spray it with nonstick cooking spray. Season the halibut with salt and pepper then rub with one teaspoon of olive oil and add it to the baking dish. Bake ten to fifteen minutes or until cooked through. Fork test the fish. If it flakes, it's ready. Remove from oven and let cool.

Take the two halves of the sliced Ciabatta bread and brush the inside of them with olive oil. Place them on a baking sheet and toast them in the oven for six to eight minutes or until golden brown. Remove them and dust with garlic powder then spread the mayonnaise equally on each of the four slices of bread.

In a medium bowl add the mashed tomatoes, capers, basil, parsley, garlic and lemon zest. Flake the fish apart and add it to the bowl then stir. Spoon the mixture onto the bread. Add fresh arugula, and top with the other half of bread loaf. Cut into individual sandwiches and serve immediately.

Mediterranean-Style Grilled Salmon with Basil

Salmon is an extremely nutritious fish that contains vitamins B12, B6, B3, vitamin D, selenium, protein, phosphorus, omega 3 fatty acids, choline, pantothenic acid, biotin, and potassium. The omega-3 fatty acids help control inflammation, maintain good cell functioning and reduce triglyceride levels in the blood. The lower the triglycerides levels the lower the risk of heart attacks, strokes, heart arrhythmias and blood pressure problems.

Salmon also contains selenium which reduces joint inflammation, prevents certain types of cancer and protects the cardiovascular system at the molecular level.

Serves 4

Ingredients

4 salmon fillets.....5 ounces each

Fresh basil.....4 tablespoons chopped

Fresh parsley.....1 tablespoon chopped

Garlic.....1 tablespoon minced

Lemon.....2 tablespoons lemon juice

Green olives.....4 chopped

Lemon.....4 thin slices

Black pepper.....to taste

Directions

Prepare a hot charcoal grill fire, heat a gas grill, or set the oven to a high broil.

Lightly coat the grill rack or broiler pan with cooking spray away from any heat sources. Position the cooking rack four to six inches from the heat source.

In a small bowl, combine the basil, lemon juice, minced garlic and parsley.

Place the fish on a cooking platter or foil and lightly spray with nonstick cooking spray. Sprinkle each fillet with black pepper the top with equal amounts of the basil-garlic mixture.

Place the fish herb-side down on the grill. Grill over high heat.

Prepare a piece of foil. When the salmon fillet edges turn white, after about three to four minutes it is time to flip it over. When you flip the salmon put it on the prepared foil rather than directly on the grill. Move to an area of reduced heat to cook through.

Test with a fork or knife. Fish should flake apart when cooked through. The thickest part of the fish should be at least 145 degrees on the thermometer.

Total cooking time is ten to fifteen minutes depending on the size and thickness of the salmon fillets. Transfer the salmon to plates and garnish with four lemon slices and four chopped olives.

Asparagus and Garlic Calzone with Pizza Sauce

When buying asparagus plan to use it within a couple of days or it will go bad. It has a higher respiration rate than most other vegetables which means it ripens faster and loses valuable nutrients. To keep the asparagus nice and crisp you can wrap the bottom roots with dampened paper towels to slow the respiration rate. You will still however need to use it within a couple of days in order to take advantage of the vegetables full nutritional value.

Serves 2

Ingredients

Asparagus.....3 stalks cut into 1-inch pieces

Pizza sauce.....2/3 cup

Spinach.....1/2 cup chopped

Broccoli.....1/2 cup chopped

Mushrooms.....1/2 cup sliced

Garlic.....2 tablespoons minced

Tomato.....1 medium sliced

Extra virgin olive oil.....4 teaspoons divided

Frozen whole-wheat bread dough loaf, thawed.....1/2 pound

Mozzarella cheese.....1/2 cup

Extra virgin olive oil cooking spray

Directions

Preheat the oven to 400 degrees. Lightly coat a baking sheet with cooking spray and set aside.

In a medium bowl add the asparagus, broccoli, garlic, mushrooms and spinach.

Drizzle two teaspoons of olive oil over the vegetables and toss to coat.

Heat a large, nonstick frying pan over medium-high heat. Add the vegetables tossed with olive oil and sauté for four to five minutes, stirring frequently. Remove from heat and set aside to cool.

On a floured surface, cut the bread dough in half. Form each half into a circle. Using a rolling pin, roll the dough into an oval shape. On one half of the oval shaped dough add half the vegetables, half the tomato slices and a quarter cup of cheese.

Wet your finger with a dab of water and rub the edge of the dough that has the vegetable filling on it.

Fold the dough over the filling to meet the edge of the dough on the bottom. Gently press both of the edges together and roll them to form a lip. Use a fork and press down along the outside rim sealing the edges together.

Place the calzone on the prepared baking sheet. Repeat to make the other calzone. Don't forget to add a little flour to the bottom of the breadboard surface for easier removal and transfer of the raw calzone.

Brush the calzones with the remaining two teaspoons olive oil. Bake until golden brown, about fifteen minutes.

Heat the pizza sauce in the microwave or on the stovetop. Place each calzone on a plate. Serve with one third cup pizza sauce on the side or pour the sauce over the calzones.

Chapter 5

Dinner

Don't forget to include one 5 ounce glass of red wine with your meal!

....and some fruit for dessert as Mediterranean people do!

Also, remember to buy fresh, organic foods as much as possible or grow your own and make your own pastas. This is the best way to get the most nutritional value from what you eat.

Sicilian Spaghetti with Anchovy and Garlic

If you've been feeling a little tired and out of sorts lately, this is the perfect dish for you! Anchovies have high levels of B12, niacin and riboflavin that play an important role in energy production as well as red blood cell creation.

The anchovy packs a punch in the way of flavor. It is a small fish with big flavor!

The health benefits of anchovies include lowering bad cholesterol and toxin levels, supporting heart health, reducing the risk of osteoporosis, skin health support and the maintenance of strong teeth.

Serves 8

Ingredients

Spaghetti.....1 pound

Extra virgin olive oil.....4 tablespoons

Garlic cloves.....3 crushed

Anchovy fillets.....1 2-ounce can chopped

Bread crumbs....1 cup, fine

Fresh parsley.....1 cup chopped

Parmesan cheese.....4 tablespoons freshly grated

Salt.....1 tablespoon

Black pepper.....to taste

Directions

In a large pot add a tablespoon of salt and fill the pot three quarters full of water. Bring to a boil.

Add the spaghetti and cook for another eight to ten minutes until the pasta is cooked to Al Dente.

In a medium skillet on medium heat, add the extra virgin olive oil, garlic and chopped anchovy fillets. Cook and stir for two to three minutes.

Add breadcrumbs and parsley to the skillet ingredients. Turn off the heat.

Add some black pepper to taste

Strain the cooked pasta and place it back into the large pot.

Add the skillet contents to the large pot of pasta and mix the ingredients together.

Plate and add parmesan cheese to each plate of pasta. Serve immediately.

Shrimp in White Wine with Penne Pasta

Shrimp is a great source of anti-inflammatory and antioxidant vitamins and minerals. However, too much shrimp can raise cholesterol levels.

Shrimp has a high level of selenium which is about 102 percent of the daily recommendation for medium shrimp. Due to shrimps rich nutrient astaxanthin, researches are finding new ways to lower the risk of colon cancers.

Serves 8

Ingredients

Penne pasta.....1 - 16 ounce package

Extra virgin olive oil.....2 tablespoons

Red onion.....1/4 cup chopped

Garlic.....1 tablespoon chopped

White wine.....1/4 cup

Tomatoes.....3 - 14.5 ounce can diced

Shrimp.....1 pound peeled and deveined

Parmesan cheese.....1 cup grated

Directions

Fill a large pot three quarters full of water and add one teaspoon of salt. Bring to a boil and add penne pasta. Check pasta within eight to ten minutes. The pasta will be done when it is Al Dente, meaning slightly firm.

While pasta is boiling, place a medium saucepan over medium heat and add two tablespoons of olive oil and heat.

Add chopped red onion and chopped garlic. Cook until the onions are opaque and the garlic is toasted.

Add diced tomatoes and white wine and mix well. Reduce to simmer and let the flavors marinate for ten minutes stirring occasionally.

Add the shrimp to the skillet and let the shrimp cook five to seven minutes.

Drain the pasta and return it to the large pot.

Take the cooked ingredients in the skillet and add to the large pasta pot. Mix and serve hot with grated parmesan cheese.

Mediterranean Chicken with White Wine

The extra virgin title in olive oil tells us that the olives used in the bottle were pressed one time during the processing stage of the olive oil. Extra virgin olive oil therefore has a higher level of nutrients that is healthier than olive oils that were pressed many times and don't have the words "extra virgin" in their title.

Serves 6

Ingredients

Extra virgin olive oil.....2 tablespoons

White wine.....2 tablespoons

Chicken breast halves.....6 boneless, skinless

Garlic cloves.....3 minced

Onion.....1/2 cup diced

Tomatoes.....3 cups chopped

White wine.....1/2 cup

Fresh thyme.....2 teaspoons chopped

Fresh basil.....1 tablespoon chopped

Kalamata olives.....1/2 cup

Fresh parsley.....1/4 cup chopped

Salt.....pinch

Pepper.....to taste

Directions

In a large skillet on medium heat add the olive oil, two tablespoons of white wine, and the chicken breast. Sauté for four to six minutes on each side allowing the chicken to turn a golden brown. Remove the chicken from the skillet and set aside to return to the pan later. In the same skillet, sauté the onions and garlic for two minutes. Add the tomatoes and bring to a boil. Lower the heat to simmer and add the white wine, basil and thyme. Simmer for fifteen minutes to allow the flavors to marinate.

Return the chicken to the skillet and cook on low heat until the chicken is cooked through. Add olives, parsley, salt and pepper. Plate and serve immediately.

Garlic Linguine

Did you know that garlic is part of the lily family along with onions and leeks? Garlic can help our bodies break down iron at the cellular level allowing the iron to disperse to other areas of the body that need the nutrients most. The sulfide in garlic also assists with blood vessel dilation keeping blood pressure under control. It helps to lower blood triglycerides which aid in lower cholesterol levels.

Serves 4

Ingredients

Linguine.....8 ounces

Tomatoes.....2 cups chopped

Garlic.....2 teaspoons, minced

Basil.....1 tablespoon, dried

Thyme.....1 teaspoon, dried

Oregano.....1 tablespoon, dried

Fresh Parsley.....2 tablespoons chopped

Extra virgin olive oil.....2 tablespoons

Directions

Fill a large pasta pot three quarters full of water and boil.

Add pasta to the boiling water and cook until it reaches your desired level of tenderness.

Add olive oil to a large saucepan over medium heat.

Add the garlic, basil, oregano and thyme to the saucepan and stir. When the linguine is cooked, add it to the large saucepan with the garlic and herbs. Mix well. Add the tomatoes and stir until the ingredients are well mixed.

Remove from heat. Top with fresh parsley and serve immediately.

Salmon Panzanella with Capers and Olives

Serves 4

Ingredients

Kalamata olives.....8 pitted and chopped

Red wine vinegar.....3 tablespoons

Capers.....1 tablespoon rinsed and chopped

Tomatoes.....2 cut into 1 inch pieces

Cucumber.....1 medium peeled and seeded, cut into 1 inch slices

Red onion.....1 thinly sliced

Black pepper..... 1/2 teaspoon divided

Extra virgin olive oil.....3 tablespoons

Whole grain bread.....3 thick slices toasted, cut into one inch cubes

Fresh basil.....1/2 cup chopped

Salmon.....1 pound skinned and cut into four sections

Salt.....1/2 teaspoon

Directions

Preheat the oven to 300 degrees or prepare the grill.

In a bowl, whisk together the pitted Kalamata olives, red wine vinegar, capers and half the black pepper. Slowly whisk in the olive oil. Add the toasted and cubed bread, cucumbers, tomatoes, onion and basil.

Oil the grill or baking dish to avoid sticking.

Season both sides of the salmon with the remaining black pepper and salt. Broil or grill the salmon for about five minutes on each side until the fish fillet flakes.

Gently mix the ingredients in the bowl and place on individual serving platters. Top with broiled or grilled fish fillets and serve immediately.

Herbed Lamb Chops with Greek Couscous Salad

Lamb chops are very nutritious. Choose organic lamb chops and ask for 100% grass fed meat for the best quality.

Organic lamb contains vitamin B3, protein, selenium, B12, zinc and phosphorus.

Serves 4

Ingredients

Lamb chops.....8 - fat trimmed off

Feta cheese.....1/2 cup crumbled

Cucumber.....1 medium peeled and chopped

Tomatoes.....2 medium chopped

Whole wheat couscous.....1/2 cup

Water.....1 cup

Fresh dill.....2 tablespoons finely chopped

Lemon.....1 for 3 tablespoons lemon juice

Extra virgin olive oil.....2 teaspoons

Fresh parsley.....1 tablespoon chopped

Garlic.....2 tablespoons minced

Salt.....1/2 teaspoon

Directions

Salad:

In a medium saucepan boil one cup of water. Add couscous. When water returns to a boil reduce the heat to simmer and cover with a tight sealing lid for two minutes. Remove from the heat and let stand for another five minutes. Transfer couscous to a medium bowl and add tomatoes, cucumber, feta cheese, lemon juice, and the finely chopped dill. Stir to combine the ingredients and place in the refrigerator.

Lamb chops:

In a small bowl combine the garlic, parsley and salt. Stir together then press onto both sides of the lamb chops.

In a large skillet on medium heat add the olive oil. Let the olive oil warm, then place the seasoned lamb chops in the skillet. Cook for six to seven minutes each side.

Plate some of the couscous salad and place a lamb chop on top. Serve immediately.

Salmon Bake with Capers and Olives

Capers come from the *Capparis Spinosa* plant that is a prickly perennial native to the Mediterranean region. Capers are the unripened flower buds of this plant that are harvested, dried in the sun then pickled in vinegar, wine or brine. The curing process brings out their tangy lemon flavor. The use of capers dates back to 1200 B.C.E.

Serves 4

Ingredients

Salmon fillets.....4 skinless, about 6 ounce each

Extra virgin olive cooking spray

Cherry tomatoes.....2 cups halved

Zucchini.....1/2 cup finely chopped

Capers.....2 tablespoons, not drained

Extra virgin olive oil.....1 tablespoon

Black olives.....1 can pitted, sliced, drained (about 2 1/4 ounce can)

Salt and pepper.....to taste

Directions

Preheat the oven to 425 degrees.

Sprinkle both sides of the salmon with salt and pepper.

Spray a baking dish with cooking spray. Place the seasoned salmon in a single layer on the sprayed baking dish.

In a bowl add tomatoes, zucchini, capers, olive oil and sliced olives. Stir to combine, then spoon the mixture over the salmon in the baking dish.

Bake the salmon for twenty minutes or until the fish flakes with a fork. Plate and serve immediately.

Pasta Extravaganza with Shrimp and Kalamata Olives

Did you know that olives are actually a fruit? They are part of the drupe family of fruits. Drupes are fruits that have a meaty fiber surrounding a pit. Other drupes include mangos, cherries, peaches, and plumbs. Kalamata olives come from the city of Kalamata, Greece.

The olive *(Olea europaea)* has been cultivated in the Mediterranean region for a very long time. Since olives and olive oil are prominent in Mediterranean cuisine it is estimated that almost half of the fat consumed in the region comes from olives.

Serves 4

Ingredients

Garlic cloves.....2 minced

Shrimp.....1 pound medium, peeled and deveined

Plum tomatoes.....2 cups chopped

Fresh basil.....1/4 cup thinly sliced

Kalamata olives.....1/3 cup pitted, chopped

Capers.....2 tablespoons drained

Freshly ground black pepper.....1/4 teaspoon

Angel hair whole grain pasta..... 4 cups cooked (about 8 ounces, uncooked)

Feta cheese.....1/4 cup crumpled

Extra virgin olive oil.....2 teaspoons

Directions

In a large pot cook the angel hair whole grain pasta as per the package directions.

Add olive oil and garlic to a large nonstick skillet placed on medium heat. Sauté the garlic for a minute then add the shrimp. Sauté for another minute then add tomato and basil. Reduce heat and simmer for three minutes or until the tomato is tender.

Stir in Kalamata olives, capers and black pepper.

In a large bowl combine the Mediterranean shrimp with the pasta and stir.

Place on serving platters and crumble feta cheese over each dish. Serve immediately.

Greek Salmon Burgers with Panko and Feta

These Greek salmon burgers include an ingredient called Panko. Panko is a premade bread crumb mix that people in Italy use for deep frying ingredients. Panko uses breads with the crusts removed. The bread is torn and then has the moisture baked out of it. Nutrients in panko are equivalent to the bread used to make the panko. You can normally find Panko made with whole wheat breads. Panko is different from standard breadcrumbs in that the torn bread pieces are usually larger in Panko than in typical bread crumbs. This makes for a crispier crust when frying cutlets and similar meats.

Serves 4

Ingredients

Salmon fillets.....1 pound skinless cut into 2 inch pieces

Panko.....1/2 cup

Egg white.....1 large

Cucumber slices.....1/2 cup

Feta cheese.....1/4 cup crumbled

Ciabatta rolls.....4 (2.5 ounces) toasted

Black pepper.....1/4 teaspoon

Salt.....pinch

Directions

In a food processor, add the salmon fillet pieces, panko and one large egg white. Pulse the food processor until the salmon is finely chopped and the ingredients are well mixed.

Heat the grill or skillet to medium heat and form the salmon into four-inch patties. Put the patties on the grill or in the skillet. Season the salmon burgers with salt and pepper.

Cook five to seven minutes then flip the salmon burger. Cook an additional five to seven minutes longer and place on a toasted Ciabatta roll.

Enjoy with crumbled feta cheese and cucumbers placed on top.

Serve immediately. Enjoy!

Mediterranean Sautéed Shrimp, Fennel and Fire-Roasted Tomatoes

Fennel belongs to the *Umbelliferae* family of vegetables making it a relative of carrot, parsley, dill and coriander. One of the most amazing things about fennel is its ability to prevent the occurrence of cancer. It also has strong anti-inflammatory properties as well.

It may surprise you to know that fennel works at the cellular level to shut down a tumor cells signaling process. By shutting this system down it prevents the activation of gene alteration and triggered inflammation. Fennel also helps to protect the liver from toxic chemical injury. It is also a great source of vitamin C.

This dish is another delicious Mediterranean meal that is jam-packed with nutrients. Enjoy!

Serves 4

Ingredients

Extra-virgin olive oil.....1 tablespoon

Fennel bulb.....1 large cored, cut into 2 inch long strips (about 4 cups)

Tomatoes.....1 - 15-ounce can diced, fire-roasted brand

Fresh oregano.....1 tablespoon chopped

Shrimp.....1 pound peeled and deveined (21 to 25 shrimp per pound)

Capers.....2 tablespoons rinsed

Feta cheese.....1/4 cup crumbled

Black pepper.....1/4 teaspoon

Directions

In a large skillet over medium heat, add olive oil and strips of fennel.

Cook the fennel for six to eight minutes until golden brown, stir occasionally.

Add tomatoes and oregano to the browned fennel. Cook about thirty minutes scraping the sides.

Add the shrimp and stir occasionally. Cook the shrimp for about four minutes or until it is cooked through.

Add capers and black pepper. Stir then remove from heat. Plate the shrimp mixture and sprinkle feta cheese on top before serving.

Pan Seared Salmon with Dill Sauce, Fennel and Red Wine

Dill is native to the Mediterranean region. It helps to protect against free radicals and carcinogens and is an excellent source of calcium, iron, magnesium and dietary fiber.

Serves 4

Ingredients

Tomato.....1 large chopped

Fennel.....1 cup finely chopped, (about 1/2 bulk stalks, trimmed)

Red onion.....2 tablespoons chopped

Dill....2 tablespoons minced

Red-wine vinegar.....1 tablespoon

Salt.....1/2 teaspoon divided

Salmon fillet.....1 pound skinned

Extra virgin olive oil.....2 tablespoons

Fresh ground pepper, to taste

Directions

In a medium bowl, combine the chopped tomatoes, chopped fennel, chopped red onion, minced dill, red-wine vinegar and a dash of salt.

Cut salmon fillets into four portions. Sprinkle the front and back of the fillets with remaining salt and pepper.

In a medium skillet on high heat, add the olive oil. It should be shimmering but not smoking.

Add the salmon skin side up and brown, (about three to five minutes) then turn over to brown the other side. Remove the pan from the heat and allow the salmon to continue to cook through (about three to five minutes)

Plate the salmon and top with the salsa. Serve immediately.

Chapter 6

Side Dishes

Mediterranean side dishes often include staples like whole grains and vegetables. These side dishes are loaded with nutrients. Be creative and change up your side dishes often in order to consume a wide variety of foods regularly.

Insalata Caprese

Basil is high in vitamin K amd also provides manganese, copper, vitamins A, C, calcium, iron, folate and magnesium. This fresh herb provides nutrients that are essential for the cardiovascular system. It protects the lining of body structures such as the blood vessel system and helps to prevent free radical damage in the bloods system itself. Vitamin K also protects against the development of blood clots. It also supports bone health and is required for the activation of osteocalcin.

Serves 6

Ingredients

Tomatoes.....4 large sliced 1/4 inch thick

Mozzarella cheese.....1 pound sliced 1/4 inch thick

Fresh basil leaves.....1/3 cup

Extra virgin olive oil.....3 tablespoons

Black pepper.....to taste

Salt.....to taste

Directions

Using a large platter, arrange the tomatoes, mozzarella cheese slices and basil leaves alternating all three as they overlap one another.

Add salt and pepper to taste. Serve immediately or wrap with plastic wrap and chill for fifteen minutes before serving.

Mediterranean Kale

One of the healthiest ways to cook kale is in a steamer. When using a double broiler, Kale only needs five-minutes of steam to make your Mediterranean diet meal pop with flavor!

Eating Kale raw is the best way to retain its nutrients. Kales most abundant nutrient is easy to remember – it's Vitamin K! One cup of Kale contains 1180.1% of our DRI (dietary reference intakes) of vitamin K. It also provides 590.2% of our DRI of vitamin A and 71% or our DRI of vitamin C.

Serves 6

Ingredients

Kale.....12 cups chopped

Lemon.....1 - 2 tablespoons lemon juice

Extra virgin olive oil.....1 tablespoon or as needed

Garlic.....1 tablespoon minced

Soy sauce.....1 teaspoon

Salt and pepper.....to taste

Directions

Using a steamer, fill the lower half of the pan with water and place on high heat. Bring the water to a boil.

In a strainer, clean and rinse the kale then place it in the top part of the steamer

Insert the basket of kale into the steamer and place the lid on top for five minutes.

In a medium bowl, add olive oil, soy sauce, lemon juice, minced garlic, salt and black pepper. Whisk the ingredients together then add the steamed kale. Stir to blend. Serve.

Sautéed Spinach with Pine Nuts, Parmesan and Golden Raisins

Spinach contains a long list of nutrients. Vitamin K, vitamin A, manganese, folate, and magnesium are the top five nutrients in spinach. Vitamin K aids blood flow and supports anti-clotting processes.

Carotenoids, beta-carotene, lutein and zeaxanthin are all provided by the Vitamin A in spinach. Vitamin A also aids in cancer prevention if eaten regularly.

Manganese aids in bone health, blood sugar control and maintaining good antioxidant levels.

Folate aids in red blood cell production, allows nerves to function correctly, aids in skin cell health, prevents homocysteine from building in the blood, aids muscular fatigue and more.

Magnesium is similar to folate and supports bone health, energy production, controls inflammation and enhances blood sugar control factors.

Serves 2

Ingredients

Extra virgin olive oil.....2 teaspoons

Golden raisins.....2 tablespoons

Pine nuts.....1 tablespoon

Garlic cloves.....2 minced

Fresh spinach.....10 ounces

Balsamic vinegar.....2 teaspoons

Fresh parmesan cheese.....1 tablespoon shaved

Fresh ground pepper.....to taste

Salt.....1/2 teaspoon

Directions

Heat the olive oil in a large nonstick skillet on medium high heat. Add garlic, raisins and pine nuts. Cook for about one minute and add spinach. Stir and cook until the spinach wilts, about two minutes.

Remove from heat and add vinegar, salt and pepper. Serve immediately with the shaved parmesan cheese on the side.

Add fresh ground pepper to taste.

Butternut Squash Pilaf

Butternut squash is a winter squash. Winter Squash contains Vitamins A, B6, B2, B3, C, K, fiber, manganese, copper, potassium, folate, pantothenic acid, omega-3, and magnesium. One cup of this summer squash and you will get 535.36 mcg RAE.

There are two types of Vitamin A. One type is in animal foods and the other type is in plant foods. The butternut squash in the plant food variety offers nutrients rich in carotenoids. Most of these act as an anti-inflammatory or antioxidant.

Serves 8

Ingredients

Butternut squash.....2 pounds peeled, halved, and seeded

Extra virgin olive oil.....1 tablespoon

Red onion.....1 finely chopped

Garlic clove.....1 minced

Water.....2 tablespoons

Tomato paste.....1 tablespoon

Brown rice.....1 cup parboiled

Vegetable broth.....1 - 14 ounce can of vegetable broth

White wine.....1/2 cup

Fennel fronds.....1/2 cup chopped

Oregano.....2 tablespoons chopped

Cinnamon.....dash

Black pepper.....to taste

Salt.....1/2 teaspoon

Directions

Grate butternut squash through the large holes of a box grater.

In a cast iron skillet heat the olive oil to medium heat.

Add the red onion and garlic clove. Stir to mix. Allow the onion to turn opaque, about ten minutes.

In a small bowl add two tablespoons of water and the tomato paste. Mix and transfer to the skillet of onions and garlic.

Add parboiled brown rice and stir to coat.

Slowly add the butternut squash and allow the squash to reduce down making enough room to cover with the lid. Increase the heat to medium high and add the broth.

Add the wine to the skillet. Cover and bring to a boil.

Reduce the heat to medium low and cook covered until the rice has absorbed most of the liquid and the squash is tender, about twenty five to thirty minutes.

Add fennel fronds, oregano, cinnamon, salt and pepper. Gently stir to mix. Remove from heat and let stand for five minutes before serving.

Stuffed Roasted Red Peppers

Red peppers are in the bell pepper family. Bell peppers offer some great nutrients provided we don't destroy their nutrients in the cooking process.

One of the bell peppers highest nutritional values when eaten raw is vitamin C. One cup of bell peppers provides 156.6% of our recommended daily allowance of vitamin C.

Serves 6

Ingredients

Red bell peppers.....6 large

Extra virgin olive oil.....1 tablespoon

Garlic cloves.....4 minced

Spinach.....6 ounces

Lemon.....1 tablespoon juice

Couscous..... 3/4 cup uncooked

Feta cheese.....1/2 cup crumbled

Salt.....1 teaspoon

Directions

Gas stove - Roast on an open flame and turn with tongs. Roasting time is about two minutes.

Broiler - Roast two inches from the heat source. Turn the peppers every five minutes. Continue for about fifteen minutes or until the peppers are roasted on all sides.

After roasting the peppers, transfer them into a large bowl. Cover with plastic wrap and cool.

When the peppers have cooled, cut the top off and remove the stem. Remove the seeds from the inside.

Heat the olive oil in a sauté pan over medium heat.

Add the garlic and sauté for about a minute.

Add spinach and cook until wilted, about 2 minutes and transfer to a bowl.

Take the bowl of spinach and stir in the lemon juice then season with salt.

Preheat the oven to 350 degrees.

In a small pot, cook the couscous as directed on the package, about five minutes.

Add the couscous to the wilted spinach and top with crumbled feta cheese. Mix well.

Line a baking pan with aluminum foil. Stuff all the roasted red peppers with the couscous spinach stuffing.

Bake on the center rack for about eight minutes. Serve immediately.

Mediterranean Basmati Mint Salad

Basmati is a type of rice that originated in India. It comes in brown and white varieties. There is a nutritional difference between Basmati and other kinds of rice. Basmati offers more of the chemical 2-acetyl-1-pyrroline which emits a special aroma when cooking. Basmati brown rice also contains about twenty percent more fiber.

In terms of white rice, it has a longer shelf life than brown but brown rice has more nutrients. The white rice nutrients are reduced by more than half of the nutrients of brown rice due to the removal of the outer kernel and the polishing process used to grind the rice down to its white appearance. Brown rice retains the bran layer, germ layer and aleurone layer. These layers contain the most fat and the most nutrients of the rice grain. When suppliers remove these layers, it greatly increases their shelf life.

To obtain the most nutrients from your rice, you want all of the layers to remain on the rice so choosing a brown rice would be your best option.

Serves 4

Ingredients

Sun dried tomatoes.....2 (packed in oil)

Hot water.....1/4 cup

Basmati rice.....1 ¼ cups uncooked

Water.....2 cups

Feta cheese.....2/3 cup crumbled

Dried currants.....2 tablespoons

Fresh mint.....2 tablespoons chopped

Extra virgin olive oil.....1 tablespoon

Pine nuts.....2 tablespoons toasted

Black pepper.....1/4 teaspoon

Salt.....1/2 teaspoon

Directions

Rehydrate the tomatoes by setting them in hot water, about one fourth cup. Set aside.

Place the rice in a large bowl, cover with water at least two inches above the rice line. Place a lid on the bowl and soak for twenty minutes then drain and rinse.

In a small saucepan over medium high heat, combine the rice, salt and two cups of water. Bring to a boil and stir frequently to avoid any sticking. Boil for five minutes or until the water reduces down. Lower the heat to simmer and cook another ten minutes. Remove from heat and let cool.

Toast the pine nuts on a baking sheet. Heat the oven to 300 degrees and toast for a couple minutes.

In a medium bowl add the cool rice, feta cheese, dried currants, fresh mint, olive oil and top with toasted pine nuts. Add black pepper to taste.

Chapter 7

Salads

The combination of extra virgin olive oil and leafy green salad packs a powerful nutritional punch!

Easy Arugula Salad with Pine Nuts

Arugula has a high level of vitamin A, vitamin C, vitamin K, folate, calcium, magnesium, phosphate and zinc as well as a nutrient called myrosinase. Myrosinase helps to boost the cancer fighting nutrients in broccoli so it's a good idea to include an arugula salad with a side of broccoli.

Serves 4

Ingredients

Arugula.....4 cups rinsed and dried

Cherry tomatoes.....1 cup halved

Pine nuts.....1/4 cup

Extra virgin olive oil.....2 tablespoons

Rice vinegar.....1 tablespoon

Fresh parmesan cheese.....1/4 cup grated

Avocado.....1 large peeled, pitted and sliced

Black pepper.....to taste

Salt.....1/2 teaspoon

Directions

In a large bowl combine arugula, cherry tomatoes, pine nuts, oil, vinegar, salt, pepper and grated cheese. Stir, then dish into salad bowls. Decorate with avocado slices.

Mediterranean Style Chickpea Salad

Chickpeas belong to the legume family and are also called garbanzo beans. They reduce the risk of cardiovascular disease by reducing bad cholesterol. If you consumed ¾ cups a day of chickpeas then tested your triglyceride (a type of fat in your blood) levels after one month your triglyceride levels would have significantly decreased. This information is based on recent studies.

Serves 4

Ingredients

Garbanzo beans.....1 - 15 ounce can rinsed and drained

Roma tomato.....1 seeded and diced

Green bell pepper.....1/2 diced

Onion.....1 small finely chopped

Garlic clove.....1 minced

Fresh parsley.....1 tablespoon chopped

Extra virgin olive oil.....2 tablespoons

Lemon.....1 juiced

Directions

Combine the garbanzo beans, bell pepper, onion, tomato, garlic, parsley, olive oil and lemon juice in a medium bowl. Stir to mix ingredients.

Serve immediately or cover and chill.

Mediterranean Diet Medley Salad

The Mediterranean diet medley salad offers a nice selection of heart-healthy nutrients. Cucumber offers three different strains of lignan that aid in reducing the risk of cardiovascular disease and certain types of cancers. Cucumbers also offer flavonoids which help to protect blood vessels against rupture or leakage.

Cucumbers are also 95% water so they keep the body hydrated and assist with eliminating toxins.

This recipe allows you to choose how much of each vegetable you want in the salad.

Serves 4

Ingredients

Cucumbers..... sliced

Carrots.....chopped

Red onions.....diced

Red pepper.....diced

Green pepper.....diced

Cherry tomatoes.....halved

Zucchini.....sliced

Feta cheese.....2 ounces crumbled

Kalamata olives.....1/4 cup pitted, sliced

Fresh basil leaves.....1/2 cup torn

Extra virgin olive oil..... 2 tablespoons

Balsamic vinegar.....1 tablespoon

Salt.....pinch

Black pepper.....dash

Directions

Combine all the ingredients in a large bowl and mix together. Serve.

Warm Arugula Bread Salad

Adding fresh parmesan to your meals can give your body a boost of nutrition. Two ounces of parmesan cheese contains 20.3 grams of protein. The body uses protein to repair and maintain itself. Protein also exists in every cell of your body. Parmesan cheese is also easy to digest and is an excellent source of calcium.

Serves 4

Ingredients

Whole-wheat bread.....2 slices cut into cubes

Extra virgin olive oil.....3 tablespoons divided

Cherry tomatoes.....1 cup halved

Arugula......8 cups

Garlic.....1 tablespoon minced

Balsamic vinegar.....2 tablespoons

Fresh parmesan cheese.....1/4 cup grated

Salt.....1/8 teaspoon

Black pepper.....1/8 teaspoon

Directions

In a large skillet on medium high heat add two tablespoons of olive oil and let the oil warm for one minute. Add the bread and let it toast on all sides.

Add tomatoes and arugula. Stir and cook until arugula wilts, about one minute.

Push the mixture to one side of the skillet. Add the remaining tablespoon of olive oil on the cleared side of the skillet. Add garlic and cook until it is lightly browned and fragrant.

Mix all the ingredients together. Remove skillet from heat.

Add salt and pepper then drizzle with balsamic vinegar.

In a large bowl, transfer the ingredients and add grated parmesan cheese over top. Serve.

Greek Salad with Chicken

Chicken has an enormous amount of nutrients however you need to consider how the chicken is raised (what it is fed and if it is pasture raised), how it is cooked and what part of the chicken you are using. Pasture raised organic chicken offers vitamins B3, B6, B12, protein, selenium, phosphorus, choline and pantothenic acid.

Serves 4

Ingredients

Chicken.....2 ½ cups, cooked and chilled (about 12 ounces)

Romaine lettuce.....6 cups, chopped

Tomatoes.....2 chopped

Cucumber.....1 medium, chopped

Red wine vinegar.....1/3 cup

Black olives.....1/2 cup pitted and sliced

Feta cheese.....1/2 cup

Red onion.....1/2 cup finely chopped

Fresh dill or oregano.....1 tablespoon chopped

Garlic powder.....1 teaspoon

Extra virgin olive oil.....2 tablespoons

Salt.....1/4 teaspoon

Pepper.....1/4 teaspoon

Directions

In a large bowl whisk together the red wine vinegar, olive oil, dill or oregano, salt pepper and garlic powder.

Add lettuce, tomatoes, cucumbers, onions, olives, cooked chicken and feta cheese. Stir together and serve on chilled plates.

Braised Kale with Cherry Tomatoes and Garlic

Garlic contains antioxidants that can boost your immune system and improve your skin. It also supports the respiratory and circulatory system and prevents inflammation due to the anti-inflammatory properties that it contains.

Serves 4

Ingredients

Kale.....1 pound, hard stems removed, chopped coarsely

Extra-virgin olive oil.....2 teaspoons

Garlic cloves.....4 thinly sliced

Vegetables stock or chicken broth.....1/2 cup

Cherry tomatoes.....1 cup halved

Lemon.....1 tablespoon lemon juice

Black pepper.....1/8 teaspoon

Directions

Heat the olive oil and garlic in a large pan on medium heat. Sauté until the garlic is lightly toasted, about 1 or 2 minutes.

Add the kale, vegetable stock or chicken broth and cover to simmer.

Lower the heat to medium low and cook until the kale wilts, about five minutes.

Remove the lid, add the tomatoes and cook until the kale is tender.

Transfer the kale to a medium bowl and add the lemon juice salt and pepper. Serve immediately.

Beet Walnut Apple Salad

To serve great tasting beets that are high in nutrition try steaming them for fifteen minutes or bake them for less than an hour. Beets offer antioxidants, anti-inflammatory benefits, cell detox benefits, as well as a whole slew of other nutrients that our bodies need daily.

Serves 8

Ingredients

Beets.....1 small bunch equal to 3 cups

Red-wine vinegar.....1/4 cup

Apple.....1/4 cup chopped

Celery.....1/4 cup chopped

Balsamic vinegar.....3 tablespoons

Extra virgin olive oil.....1 tablespoon

Water.....1 tablespoon

Fresh salad greens.....8 cups

Walnuts.....3 tablespoons chopped

Gorgonzola cheese.....1/4 cup crumbled

Freshly ground black pepper

Directions

Steam the raw beets in a saucepan until tender. Slip the skins off. Rinse to cool and slice into half inch rounds.

Toss the beets with the red wine vinegar in a medium bowl.

Add apples and celery and combine.

In a large bowl combine the balsamic vinegar, olive oil and water.

Add the salad greens and toss.

Put the greens onto individual salad plates. Top with the beet mixture. Sprinkle with pepper, walnuts and cheese. Serve immediately.

Rainbow Greek Salad

Tomatoes contain antioxidants that support bone, liver, kidney and blood health. Tomatoes also help regulate fats in the bloodstream and reduce the risk of heart disease with their antioxidant properties. Cancer research has shown that tomatoes can also lower the risk of prostate cancer as well as some lung cancers, pancreatic cancer and breast cancer.

Serves 6

Ingredients

Tomatoes.....3 large chopped

Cucumbers.....2 peeled and chopped

Red onion.....1 small chopped

Extra virgin olive oil.....1/4 cup

Lemon.....1 - 4 teaspoons of lemon juice

Oregano......1 ½ teaspoons

Feta cheese.....1 cup crumbled

Black Kalamata olives.....6 pitted and sliced

Salt and pepper....to taste

Directions

In a deep platter or shallow bowl add tomatoes, onion, cucumbers, oil, lemon juice and oregano. Season with salt and pepper.

Top with feta cheese and Kalamata olives. Serve.

Roasted Red Pepper with Feta Salad

Basil is one of the oldest and most popular herbs. It is extremely rich in phytonutrients and is referred to as a "holy herb" in many countries. Basil contains very high levels of vitamin A, beta-carotene, lutein, zea-xanthin and cryptoxanthin. These compounds help protect against free radical damage. 100 grams of basil contains a surprising 175 % of the daily required dose of vitamin A.

Serves 4

Ingredients

Fat-free feta cheese.....1/4 cup

Fat-free blue cheese dressing.....2 tablespoons

Whole roasted red peppers.....2 divided in half and cut into strips

Extra virgin olive oil.....4 tablespoons

Fresh Basil.....2 tablespoons plus four leaves for garnish

Freshly ground black pepper.....to taste

Directions

Combine the blue cheese dressing and feta cheese together in a small bowl.

Arrange half a red pepper in the center of four small serving plates. Drizzle each serving with one teaspoon of olive oil and one tablespoon of the feta cheese-blue cheese mixture. Sprinkle with black pepper and half a tablespoon of basil. Garnish each with a basil leaf and serve at room temperature.

Chapter 8

Fruity Sweet Snacks

Fruit is a staple on the Mediterranean diet so feel free to have fun with it! The great thing about the Mediterranean diet is that it encourages you to eat a variety of foods in moderation. That includes sweets!

As long as you adhere to the Mediterranean diet pyramids suggested serving of sweets you're good to go!

Avocado and Tuna Tapas

The word *Tapas* means small Spanish savory foods such as appetizers or snacks that are typically served with drinks in a bar style setting.

Avocado is actually a fruit, not a vegetable. It is a superfood that provides an array of health benefits. Avocados are loaded with carotenoids. They can help you lose weight, stabilize blood sugar and lower cholesterol.

Tuna is packed with selenium, vitamin B3, B6, B12, protein, phosphorus, vitamin B1, B2, D, choline, potassium and magnesium.

Serves 4

Ingredients

Solid white tuna packed in water..... 1 - 12 ounce can drained

Homemade mayonnaise.....1 tablespoon (recipe below)

Green onions.....3 sliced, plus stalks for garnish

Red pepper.....1/2 chopped

Balsamic vinegar.....1 dash

Avocados.....2 ripe halved and pitted

Black pepper.....to taste

Salt.....1/2 teaspoon

Directions

Homemade mayonnaise

Makes 3/4 cups of mayo

Egg.....1 large, yolk only

Lemon.....1 – juice only, 1 ½ teaspoons

White wine vinegar.....1 teaspoon

Dijon mustard.....1/4 teaspoon

Olive oil.....3/4 cup

Avocado and Tuna Tapas

Combine all the ingredients in a medium bowl. Whisk until blended.

Add one quarter cup of the olive oil to the bowl a few drops at a time. Slowly add the remaining half cup of olive oil whisking constantly.

Cover and put in refrigerator. Keep chilled.

In a medium bowl, add tuna, mayonnaise, red pepper, green onions and balsamic vinegar. Stir together and mix well.

Season the tuna mixture with salt and pepper.

Fill the avocado halves with the tuna mixture. Use the remaining green onions to garnish.

Almond and Apricot Biscotti

Almonds support brain and bone health, increase good cholesterol and decrease bad cholesterol, support the immune system, reduce inflammation, regulate blood pressure, boost energy and help to prevent cancer.

Makes 24 cookies

Ingredients

Whole-wheat flour.....1 ½ cups

Brown sugar.....1/4 cup firmly packed

Baking powder.....1 teaspoon

1 percent low-fat milk.....2 tablespoons

Eggs.....2 beaten

Walnut oil.....2 tablespoons

Dark honey.....2 tablespoons

Almond extract.....1/2 teaspoon

Dried apricots.....2/3 cup chopped

Almonds.....1/4 cup coarsely chopped

Directions

Preheat the oven to 350 degrees.

In a large bowl combine the flour, baking powder and brown sugar. Whisk to blend. Add the milk, eggs, walnut oil, honey and almond extract. Stir until the dough begins to come together. Add the chopped apricots and almonds. With floured hands, mix until the dough is well blended.

Place the dough on a long sheet of plastic wrap and shape by hand into a flattened log twelve inches long, three inches wide and about one inch high. Lift the plastic wrap to invert the dough onto a nonstick baking sheet. Bake until lightly brown, about 20 minutes. Transfer to another baking sheet to cool for five minutes. Leave the oven set at 350 degrees.

Place the cooled log on a cutting board. With a serrated knife, cut crosswise on the diagonal into 24 slices half an inch wide. Arrange the slices, cut-side down on the baking sheet. Return to the oven and bake until crisp, fifteen to twenty minutes. Transfer to a wire rack and let them cool completely.

Berries Marinated in Balsamic Vinegar

Strawberries contain vitamin B6, vitamin C, manganese, fiber, iodine, folate, copper, potassium, biotin, phosphorus, magnesium, and omega 3 fats. Blueberries contain vitamin C, manganese, vitamin K, fiber and copper.

Raspberries include vitamin C, manganese, fiber, copper, vitamin K, pantothenic acid, biotin, vitamin E, magnesium, folate, omega 3 fats and potassium. The vinegar in this dish will help to keep the fruit fresh.

Just cleaning your berries in a little water and vinegar when you bring them home will kill any mold spores on the fruit.

Serves 2

Ingredients

Balsamic vinegar.....1/4 cup

Brown sugar.....2 tablespoons

Vanilla extract.....1 teaspoon

Strawberries.....1/2 cup sliced

Blueberries.....1/2 cup

Raspberries.....1/2 cup

Shortbread biscuits.....2

Directions

Whisk together the balsamic vinegar, brown sugar and vanilla in a small bowl.

In another bowl, add the raspberries, strawberries and blueberries. Pour the balsamic vinegar mixture over the berries. Let the fruit marinate for ten to fifteen minutes. Drain the marinade. Refrigerate or serve immediately.

To serve, divide the berries into two serving dishes and place the shortbread biscuit on the side of each bowl.

Frosty Almond Date Shake

Pitted dates contain calcium, iron, vitamin B, vitamin K and folate. Dates are a great source of phenols and antioxidants which protect cells against free radicals.

Serves 4

Ingredients

Fresh Dates.....1/3 cup pitted and chopped

Water....2 tablespoons warm

Vanilla almond milk.....2 cups chilled

Plain Greek yogurt.....1/2 cup

Banana.....1 very ripe frozen

Ice cubes.....4

Ground nutmeg.....1/8 teaspoon plus extra for garnish

Directions

In a small bowl add the chopped dates and sprinkle with the warm water. Let soak for five minutes to soften and then drain or pat dry with a paper towel.

In a blender, combine the yogurt, almond milk, banana, dates, ice cubes and one eighth teaspoon of nutmeg. Blend until smooth and frothy, about thirty seconds.

Pour into tall, chilled glasses and garnish each with a dusting of nutmeg.

Strawberries with Minted Yogurt

The maximum time that you can store strawberries and retain their vitamin C levels is only two days. Losing the vitamin C means that you also lose valuable polyphenol antioxidants. It is best to store them in the storage bins of your refrigerator as they provide additional humidity.

Serves 4

Ingredients

Plain Greek yogurt.....1/2 cup

Buttermilk.....1/2 cup

Sugar.....1 tablespoon

Fresh mint.....1 ½ teaspoons chopped

Vanilla extract......1/8 teaspoon

Strawberries.....3 cups sliced

Directions

In a medium bowl, add yogurt, buttermilk, mint, sugar and vanilla. Whisk the ingredients until creamy smooth.

Slice the strawberries into four individual bowls and spoon the minty yogurt over the strawberries. Serve immediately.

Baby Tiramisu

Ricotta cheese is high in calcium and supports eye health via the vitamin A nutrients. Ricotta cheese also aids in white blood cell reproduction and cell formation. It also has trace amounts of folate, niacin, vitamin D and vitamin K.

Serves 6

Ingredients

Non-fat ricotta cheese.....1/2 cup

Confectioners' sugar.....2 tablespoons

Vanilla extract.....1/2 teaspoon

Ground cinnamon.....1/8 teaspoon

Ladyfingers..... 6

Brewed espresso or strong coffee.....4 tablespoons divided

Bittersweet chocolate chips.....2 tablespoons melted

Directions

In a large bowl, combine sugar, vanilla, cinnamon and ricotta cheese.

In a 9 x 5 inch pan place six ladyfingers on the bottom. Drizzle two tablespoons of espresso or strong coffee over the ladyfingers. Add a layer of ricotta cheese over the coffee. Add another layer of the ladyfingers, drizzle the last of the coffee and melted chocolate.

Refrigerate until chocolate sets, about twenty minutes.

Home-Made Trail Mix

The wonderful thing about creating your own trail mix is that you can choose what nutrients you want to put into it to make your perfect blend. For this recipe you will use almonds, peanuts, cranberries, dates and dried apricots etc. Apricots are a great source of fiber and they also contain vitamin A, vitamin C and iron.

Avoid sugar-coated fruits and vegetables. Normally fruits create their own sugar so adding more is unnecessary. Buying organic is also recommended.

Serves 5

Ingredients

Almonds.....1/4 cup whole, shelled, unpeeled

Peanuts.....1/4 cup unsalted, dry-roasted

Dried cranberries......1/4 cup

Dates.....1/4 cup pitted, chopped

Dried apricots or other dried fruit.....2 ounces

Directions

In a medium bowl, combine your chosen fruits and nuts and gently stir with a large spoon. Keep in a sealed freezer bag or serve immediately. If you have a dehydrator, you can dry your own fruit for this recipe.

Blueberries with Lemon Cream

Blueberries add strength to the body's natural ability to produce stronger antioxidants when eaten regularly.

Serves 4

Ingredients

Reduced-fat cream cheese.....4 ounces

Greek vanilla yogurt.....3/4 cup

Honey.....1 teaspoon

Freshly grated lemon zest.....2 teaspoons

Fresh blueberries..... 2 cups

Directions

Break up the cream cheese with a fork in a medium bowl.

When opening the yogurt, only lift the sealed tab slightly so you can drain off any excess liquid. When the excess liquid is gone, remove the foil sealed around the container and add three quarter cups of yogurt to the medium bowl.

Add honey to the bowl and use a hand held mixer to blend the ingredients together. Beat at high speed until creamy and smooth. Add the lemon zest and continue to blend until mixed.

Plate the blueberries and the lemon zest in some dessert dishes.

Serve immediately or cover and refrigerate.

Cherries with Ricotta and Toasted Almonds

This snack will help to increase your calcium levels with the ricotta and work to reduce poor cholesterol levels at the same time. Almonds vitamin B2, provide biotin, vitamin E, manganese, copper and more. Cherries contain melatonin which is a hormone that lowers the body temperature and thus makes you sleepy. The more tart the cherries the deeper your sleep.

Serves 1

Ingredients

Cherries.....3/4 cup pitted frozen

Partly skimmed ricotta.....2 tablespoons

Slivered almonds.....1 tablespoon toasted

Directions

Warm the cherries in a microwave on high.

Top the cherries with ricotta and stir.

Sprinkle with almonds and serve.

Chapter 9

Appetizers

I absolutely love appetizers! They're cute little packages that contain bite-sized bursts of flavor and nutrients!

Lima Bean Spread with Cumin and Herbs

Lima beans are full of fiber and have a high level of molybdenum. Molybdenum is an essential mineral that jump starts the enzymes in our bodies.

Cilantro is a popular herb on the Mediterranean diet that is also called coriander. Cilantro contains numerous plant derived chemical compounds that have disease prevention and health boosting benefits.

Makes about 1 to 1 ½ cups

Ingredients

Lima beans.....10 ounces

Garlic cloves.....4 peeled and crushed

Red pepper.....1/4 cup crushed

Extra-virgin olive oil.....2 tablespoons

Lemon.....1 - 4 teaspoons lemon juice

Cumin.....1 teaspoon

Fresh mint.....1 tablespoon chopped

Cilantro.....1 tablespoon chopped

Dill.....1 tablespoon chopped

Black pepper.....to taste

Salt.....1/2 teaspoon

Directions

Fill a large saucepan three quarters full of water. Place on medium high heat and bring to a boil.

Add lima beans, red pepper and garlic. Cook until the beans are tender, about 10 minutes. Remove from heat. Do NOT drain. Let the beans set for another ten minutes then drain.

Transfer the beans to a food processor.

Add lemon, olive oil, cumin and salt and pepper. Process for several minutes until the mixture is nice and smooth. Transfer to dip bowl and add mint, cilantro and dill.

Orzo Pilaf with Mint

Orzo is a type of pasta that looks like rice or barley. Mint (either peppermint or spearmint) contains manganese, copper and vitamin C. Peppermint has relieved indigestion and stomach problems for years due to the muscle relaxing properties it contains.

Serves 8

Ingredients

Chicken broth.....6 cups reduced sodium

Extra-virgin olive oil.....1 tablespoon

Onion.....1 large, diced

Orzo.....2 cups

Fresh mint.....1/3 cup chopped

Freshly ground black pepper.....to taste

Directions

In a large saucepan over medium heat simmer the six cups of chicken broth.

In a large deep skillet over medium heat add the olive oil and onion. Cook until the onion turns opaque.

Add orzo to the skillet of onion and stir constantly for about five minutes or until the orzo is toasted.

Add one cup of the hot broth to the skillet and allow the orzo to absorb the broth. Reduce the heat to a continuous simmer. When broth is absorbed, add another cup. Continue this process until all the broth is used and the orzo is tender yet firm. The process should take fifteen to twenty minutes.

Season with salt and pepper then stir in the mint. Serve immediately.

Greek Appetizer Flat Bread

Serves 6

Ingredients

Whole grain pizza crust .....1 - 13.8 ounce can

Greek seasoning or dried oregano leaves......2 teaspoons

Fat-free cream cheese.....3 ounces softened

Fresh baby spinach leaves.....1 cup

Red onion.....1/2 cup thinly sliced

Kalamata olives.....1/3 cup pitted and cut in half

Cherry tomatoes.....6 cut in fourths

Extra virgin olive oil cooking spray

Directions

Preheat the oven to 400 degrees. Spray the bottom and sides of a 15 x 10 inch pan with cooking spray.

Unroll the dough and place it in the center of the pan. Press until the dough covers the bottom and sides of the pan evenly.

Bake the dough for thirteen to eighteen minutes. The edges of the dough should be golden brown.

In a small bowl add the dried oregano or Greek seasoning and the softened cream cheese. Stir together with a fork until mixed.

When the crust is baked, remove from oven and spread the cream cheese and Greek seasoning evenly over the crust.

Coat the top of the cheese with spinach leaves, red onions, Kalamata olives and cherry tomatoes.

Cut six rows by four rows and serve warm.

Warm Olives with Rosemary and Fennel Seeds

Olives of all types have a large amount of nutrients. Hydroxytyrosol is a phytonutrient in olives that is linked to cancer prevention. Hydroxytyrosol is also gaining attention as a nutrient that helps prevent bone loss.

Makes 1 cup

Ingredients

Black olives.....4 ounces

Green olives.....4 ounces

Extra virgin olive oil.....1/4 cup

Rosemary.....1 sprig

Fennel seeds.....1/4 teaspoon

Crushed red pepper.....1 pinch

Directions

In a small skillet over medium heat, add olive oil, green and black olives, sprig of rosemary, fennel seeds and a pinch of crushed red pepper. Sauté about three minutes or until olives begin to turn brown. Serve warm.

Spinach and Feta Pita Bake with Mushrooms and Tomatoes

Pita bread is actually "leavened wheat bread". Leavened in culinary terms is when you use an ingredient or agent that chemically reacts to heat, moisture or acidity to transform the ingredient. It is the same as yeast in regular breads. The nutrients in wheat bread resemble the nutrients used in Pita breads.

When buying whole-wheat bread, remember that in order to obtain all the nutrients, you must select one hundred percent whole-wheat. Choosing whole grains rather than refined grains is another important factor when choosing nutritional values.

If your wheat bread has been processed sixty percent then you lose nearly all the benefits of eating wheat bread.

Serves 6

Ingredients

Sun dried tomato pesto.....6 ounces

Whole-wheat pita bread.....6 - 6 inch

Roma tomatoes.....2 chopped

Fresh spinach.....1 bunch rinsed and chopped

Mushrooms.....4 sliced

Feta cheese.....1/2 cup

Parmesan cheese.....2 tablespoons grated

Extra-virgin olive oil.....3 tablespoons

Freshly ground black pepper.....to taste

Directions

Preheat the oven to 350 degrees. On a large baking sheet, place the whole-wheat pita bread in rows and spread the top of them with the tomato pesto.

Add the Roma tomatoes, mushrooms, spinach, feta cheese and parmesan cheese. Sprinkle extra-virgin olive oil over the top and add black pepper to taste.

Bake in the oven until the bread is crispy, about 12 minutes. Remove from the oven and cut into four quarters then transfer to a platter.

Serve warm.

Greek Saganaki

Saganaki is a Greek dish made of floured or breaded cheese fried in oil.

Feta cheese is a great source of calcium. Next to cheese, the only other food in which you can obtain more calcium per serving is milk. One serving of feta cheese provides 74% of your daily calcium intake. Calcium also helps balance blood pH levels. There are acid and alkaline levels in our blood. Calcium monitors oxygen levels in the blood to balance the acid/alkaline levels.

One other large nutrient you receive from cheese is protein. One serving of feta cheese provides 43 % of your daily value. Protein helps build strong muscles, keeps your immune system functioning correctly, maintains healthy hair, skin and nails and aids in the production of enzymes.

Serves 4

Ingredients

Egg.....1

Oregano.....1 teaspoon finely chopped

Feta cheese.....8 ounces

Whole wheat flour.....1/2 cup

Extra virgin olive oil.....2 tablespoons

Roma tomatoes.....2 large sliced

Lemon.....1 cut into wedges

Freshly ground black pepper.....to taste

Directions

Beat the egg in a shallow dish. Add the chopped oregano then set aside.

Slice the feta cheese into 2 x 3 inch slices making eight slices.

Place the flour in a shallow dish.

Add the olive oil to a medium saucepan over medium heat. Take a pinch of flour and drop it into the oil. If the oil bubbles around the flour it is ready.

Dip the feta cheese in the egg then transfer to the dish of flour. Coat both sides of the cheese with flour and transfer to the skillet of olive oil.

When both sides of the cheese are golden brown, use a slotted spatula to pick up the Saganaki and let the oil strain off into the skillet.

Place on a platter and pat dry so no oil remains.

Add sliced tomatoes to the platter and season with pepper.

Garnish with lemon wedges.

Chapter 10

Dressings, Dips and Sauces

Dressings, dips and sauces are a great way of adding nutrients to your diet. Be creative and use them with a variety of different foods!

Greek Tzatziki

Tzatziki is a Greek cucumber sauce served with grilled meats. The best cucumber for this sauce is the English variety since it is nearly seedless.

Cucumbers belong to the same plant family as melons, squash and pumpkins called the cucurbitaceae plant family. Cucumbers come in white, orange and yellow varieties.

When you place cucumber slices over your eyes you can reduce puffiness due to the cucumbers caffeic acid and water content.

The largest cucumber ever grown was in China. It was 67 inches long and 154 pounds!

Makes 5 cups

Ingredients

Greek strained yogurt - 32 ounce container low-fat

English cucumber.....1/2 with peel, grated (box grater only)

Garlic clove.....1 pressed

Lemon.....1 - 2 tablespoons lemon juice

Extra-virgin olive oil.....2 tablespoons

Lemon.....1 - 2 teaspoons lemon zest, grated

Fresh dill.....3 tablespoons chopped

Freshly ground black pepper..... 1 tablespoon

Sea salt.....1 tablespoon, divided

Directions

Grate the cucumber and transfer it to a small bowl. Add one half tablespoon of salt and let it sit so the liquid accumulates on the bottom.

Note: Do not use an automatic food processor. Use the hand held box grater for best results.

In a medium bowl, add the Greek strained yogurt. It will be thicker than standard Greek yogurt. Add the garlic, olive oil and lemon zest to the yogurt. Add dill, pepper and half a tablespoon of salt then whisk ingredients together until blended.

Next, return to the bowl of cucumber. Strain the juice from the cucumbers and pat dry with paper towels. Add the strained cucumber to the yogurt mixture and combine. Taste to make sure you have enough salt and pepper. Transfer to a serving dish. Best if chilled before serving.

Easy Greek Yogurt Cucumber Sauce

Lemons help to restore the body's pH balance, are a rich source of vitamin C and flavonoids that help fight flu's and colds and they contain high levels of vitamin C that neutralize the damaging effects of free radicals. They also have antibacterial properties that destroy harmful bacteria that can potentially cause life-threatening diseases.

Makes 2 cups

Ingredients

Plain Greek yogurt.....1 cup

Low fat sour cream.....1 cup

White vinegar.....1 teaspoon

Lemon.....1 - 1/2 teaspoon lemon juice

Cucumber.....1 small peeled, seeded and finely chopped

Green onion.....1 chopped

Garlic clove.....1 minced

Feta cheese.....1/4 cup crumbled

Oregano.....1/2 teaspoon

Lemon zest.....1/4 teaspoon

Salt and pepper.....to taste

Directions

Combine all the ingredients in a medium bowl. Stir together. Refrigerate and use as a vegetable dip, sandwich sauce or serve as a pita dip.

Greek Feta and Olive Spread with Sun-Dried Tomatoes

Tomatoes spoil quickly after they're picked primarily due to their high moisture content. Drying tomatoes removes the water, retains the flavor and nutrients and preserves the tomato.

Sun-dried tomatoes are an excellent source of antioxidants. A one cup serving of sun-dried tomatoes contains potassium, iron, protein, fiber, vitamin K, thiamin, riboflavin and niacin.

Makes 1 ½ cups

Ingredients

Feta cheese.....1 - 6 ounce package, crumbled

Extra virgin olive oil.....2 tablespoons

Lemon juice.....1 teaspoon

Garlic.....1/2 teaspoon minced

Sun-dried tomatoes.....2 ounces hydrated

Dried oregano.....1/2 teaspoon

Kalamata olives.....1 tablespoon pitted, drained and chopped

Black olives.....3 pitted olives to decorate

Directions

In a small bowl add some warm water and rehydrate the sun-dried tomatoes.

In a blender, add feta cheese, olive oil, lemon juice, oregano, garlic and the rehydrated tomatoes. Pulse the blender until all the ingredients are mix together well and have a smooth texture. Transfer the ingredients to a medium bowl.

Blend in the chopped olives and mix well. Place three olives in a row down the center of the dish to decorate.

Serve immediately or wrap in plastic and refrigerate until ready to use.

Greek Salad Dip

Red wine vinegar is made from red wine though it is non-alcoholic in its final form. It is very low in fat and low in calories and contains numerous trace nutrients.

Serves 8

Ingredients

Feta cheese.....8 ounces, crumbled

Black olives.....1 - 2.25 ounce can, pitted

Tomato.....1 seeded and chopped

Green onions.....3 finely chopped

Low Sodium Caesar salad dressing.....1/2 cup (see recipe below)

Low Sodium Caesar Salad Dressing ingredients: (Makes ¾ cups)

Extra virgin olive oil.....1/3 cup

Garlic cloves.....4 roasted

Lemon.....1 - 1 tablespoon lemon juice

Red wine vinegar.....2 tablespoons

Worcestershire sauce .....1/2 teaspoon

Directions

Low Sodium Caesar Salad Dressing:

Put all the ingredients in a jar with a tight fitting lid.

Place the lid on the jar and shake well. Use immediately over your favorite salad or refrigerate. Do not store the dressing out of the refrigerator as the olive oil and garlic mixture stored at room temperature can cause a chemical reaction that will result in food poisoning.

Greek Salad Dip directions:

In a large bowl, mix together the feta cheese, black olives, tomatoes, green onions and half a cup of the low sodium Caesar Salad Dressing.

Chill for twenty minutes and then serve immediately.

It's great served with crackers or toasted pita bread squares.

Roasted Red Pepper Dip

Makes 1 ¾ cups

Ingredients

Feta cheese.....8 ounces feta cheese

Red bell peppers.....2 roasted

Garlic clove.....1 minced

Greek plain yogurt.....1/4 cup

Cayenne pepper.....to taste

Directions

Roasted Bell Peppers:

Preheat the oven to a low broil and place the rack six to eight inches from the heat source.

Place bell peppers on a baking sheet then place the baking sheet on the appropriate oven rack keeping the oven door ajar. Watch the peppers as they toast.

After a few minutes, pull the rack out and turn the peppers with a pair of tongs then return to the heat and toast.

Continue this process until the peppers are nice and toasty all around. This should only take five to ten minutes for the whole process. When toasted, remove from baking sheet and set aside to cool. Turn the oven off.

Feta and Red Pepper Mix:

In a blender, add the feta cheese, garlic and yogurt. Pulse the blender a couple times to mix. Return to the roasted peppers and cut them into strips. Add the peppers to the blender.

Pulse the blender several times to ensure an even mixture of ingredients. Add cayenne pepper to taste.

Garlic Feta Dip

Garlic has anti-inflammatory, antibacterial, and antiviral properties.

Garlic is best stored in a dark, cool storage space. Don't store it in plastic bags. Simply leave it sitting out in a small basket or wide jar.

Makes 1 cup

Ingredients

Feta cheese.....1 cup crumbled

Low fat sour cream.....1/2 cup

Greek plain yogurt.....1/2 cup

Garlic.....2 cloves peeled

Freshly ground black pepper.....1/4 teaspoon

Salt.....1/4 teaspoon

Directions

In a blender or food processor, add yogurt, sour cream, garlic and feta cheese. Pulse the processor until the garlic is minced. Transfer the garlic feta dip into a serving dish. Season with salt and pepper.

Roasted Eggplant and Feta Dip

Eggplant season is August through October even though egglants are available year round. Eggplants are in the nightshade family like tomatoes, sweet peppers and potatoes. Eggplant skins contain a phytonutrient called nasunin. Nasunin is an antioxidant which protects the cell membranes from damage. This includes cell membranes related to the brain.

Serves 12 - 1/4 cup each

Ingredients

Eggplant.....1 medium - 1 pound

Lemon.....1 - 2 tablespoons lemon juice

Extra-virgin olive oil.....1/4 cup

Feta cheese.....1/2 cup, crumbled

Red onion.....1/2 cup finely chopped

Red pepper.....1 small finely chopped

Chili pepper.....1 small Jalapeno seeded and minced

Fresh basil.....2 tablespoons chopped

Fresh parsley.....1 tablespoon chopped

Cayenne pepper.....1/4 teaspoon or to taste

Salt......pinch

Sugar.....pinch if needed

Pita chips.....for dipping

Directions

Preheat the broiler and position the rack about six inches from the heat source.

Use a large baking pan lined with foil to cook the eggplant.

Wash the eggplant and poke it with holes to act as vents. This will cause the eggplant to steam during the baking process. I use a kabob skewer or a grilling fork to poke the holes.

Place the eggplant on the baking sheet and put it in the oven. Turn it with tongs every four or five minutes. Continue to turn and bake until the skin is charred and you can easily insert a knife into the dense part of the flesh near the stem. It should take about fifteen to twenty minutes. Transfer to a cutting board and allow it to cool.

In a medium bowl, add the lemon juice then go to the eggplant and cut it lengthwise on the breadboard. Scrape the eggplant flesh out of the skin and transfer it to the bowl with the lemon juice. Mix it together with the lemon juice to prevent eggplant discoloration later.

Add olive oil to the eggplant and stir until completely absorbed.

Add all the remaining ingredients except for the sugar.

Stir and mix all the ingredients together. Taste the mixture and test for bitterness.

If eggplant is not in season the bitterness level can change. If the mixture tastes bitter, use a pinch of sugar to reduce the bitterness.

Serve with pita chips. You can also change up the recipe by adding garlic and different seasonings.

Other books by Gina Crawford

Mediterranean Diet for Beginners

DASH Diet for Beginners

DASH Diet Cookbook

The 5:2 Diet for Beginners

5:2 Diet 30 Minute Recipes

Sugar Detox for Beginners

Sugar Free Recipes

Paleo for Beginners

Available on Amazon

Conclusion

I love Mediterranean-style cooking for its great flavors and health benefits. The Mediterranean diet is such a nutrient-rich diet that you can't eat the recommended foods without improving your health.

I hope that you enjoy these Mediterranean diet recipes as much as I do. May they help you experience greater health and vitality, weight loss and longevity!

About Gina Crawford

Understanding what it takes to live a healthy lifestyle, eat right, achieve your goal weight, and love your life shouldn't be complicated. Your time is valuable and the last thing you need is to tackle a 300 page book on how to get your health, weight, and life on track. If you're like most people, you just want the facts in bite-sized, easy to understand pieces that you can apply to your life TODAY!

My name is Gina Crawford. I am a health and "all things natural" enthusiast, author, mother, and wife. Years ago I was overweight, exhausted, unhappy, and desperately aching for a better life. One day, gruelingly tired of my situation, I started researching everything I could on health and transforming my life. I often felt overwhelmed by the amount of information and the changes I had to make, but I persevered and managed to turn my life around one book and one bite at a time.

Now I'm determined to share what I've learned in an easy, non-overwhelming, no fluff, no filler, straight to the point kind of way that will allow others to achieve maximum results in a short amount of time.

I am passionate about every book I write and my goal with each book is to make it simple and concise, yet power-packed with the necessary information you need to transform your life. I have learned first-hand the incredible value of healing ourselves with natural organic foods, natural remedies, exercise, and a positive mindset.

When I'm not writing, I love spending time with my family, cooking, walking, biking, and reading.

My hope is that my books will help you live a healthier, better, more passionate, alive life!

Happy reading!

Gina

Printed in Great Britain
by Amazon